The Handbook
of
Medical Ethics

The Handbook
of
Medical Ethics

Published by the British Medical Association
Tavistock Square, London, WC1H 9JP

This edition first published 1984
Second impression 1985
Third impression 1986

*Detailed advice on current issues, which may have been
altered by legislation, is available from the Secretariat.*

British Library cataloguing in publication data

The Handbook of medical ethics.
1. Medical ethics
I. British Medical Association
174'.2   R724

ISBN 0-7279-0111-7

Printed in Great Britain by the
University Press, Cambridge

Foreword

Since the formation of a Committee on Medical Ethics in 1849, the British Medical Association (BMA) has issued guidance on medical ethics. In 1980, reflecting the increased awareness by patients of ethical matters and a medical profession whose practise had been substantially modified by the technical advances and social change of previous years, a new version of the BMA's handbook was published. It attempted to set down in a co-ordinated form the profession's approach to its ethical responsibilities. This edition incorporates amendments to the 1981 edition, new material relevant to policy decisions of the Representative Body of the BMA, together with changes in presentation of material in certain sections.

Certain fundamental principles underly the whole of the book. We have attempted in the various sections to suggest how these should be applied in every day medical work. There is wide agreement on these principles among doctors in all countries, but, as conditions vary, we see this book mainly as a guide for doctors, medical students, and others in the United Kingdom concerned with the ethical issues which arise in the practice of medicine.

Contents

History of medical ethics

The dependence of patients upon the technical knowledge and the integrity of physicians in their dealings with patients has meant that a bond of trust between doctor and patient has always been required.

From earliest times, various legal systems have incorporated some degree of regulation of doctors. In the Code of Laws of Hammurabi (1790 BC) not only were fees regulated but also success was rewarded in accordance with the status of the patient: failure, however, was punished by mutilation.

The Hippocratic Oath (4th century BC) indicates the early concern of the profession to regulate itself by laying down basic standards of conduct, not only between the doctor and patient, but also between teacher and pupil. In the ensuing centuries the principles of Christian humanism dominated the practice of medicine. Traditions of etiquette in public and private life gradually evolved, coupled with those criteria of professional conduct which established the physician's position in society.

Towards the end of the 18th century the role of physicians in dealing with disease in individuals as well as population groups (as in the great epidemics) led to the drafting of codes of professional conduct, exemplified by that produced by Thomas Percival in Manchester in 1789. His proposals, "Medical Ethics or a Code of Institutes and Precepts adapted to the Professional Conduct of Physicians and Surgeons", published in 1803, laid the foundations for modern medical ethical standards in the UK.

The Provincial Medical and Surgical Association, formed in 1832 (which became the British Medical Association (BMA) in 1856) appointed a Committee on Medical Ethics in 1849. This formed the basis of the Central Ethical Committee of the BMA, which has played a leading role not only in establishing ethical standards for the medical profession in the UK, but also for the standards adopted for many years as the norms of conduct for doctors in much of the world.

The BMA played a large part in the establishment of the General Medical Council (GMC) under the Medical Act 1858, the purpose

9

of which was to enable the public to distinguish between the qualified and the unqualified practitioner, to which end a Medical Register was established. The GMC was given a regulatory role and, as a result of its experience in carrying out this function, found it expedient from time to time to issue guidance to all members of the profession so as to enable them to avoid actions which might lead to charges of misconduct in a professional respect.

Changing attitudes of society and the major advances in medical science at the end of the 19th and the beginning of the 20th centuries led to recognition of the need for modification of the Hippocratic Oath. This need was met by the Declaration of Geneva, formulated by the World Medical Association in 1947, supplemented by Declarations on particular aspects of medical ethics, such as those concerning therapeutic abortion, research, and torture and other inhuman or degrading treatment.

Since 1947 the increased rate of scientific discovery and its communication to the public has led to a growing need for the medical profession to be fully aware of society's views on these developments. This enables ethical guidelines to reflect and safeguard the interests and wellbeing of patients.

While other European countries' ethical systems have been codified and incorporated in national civil and criminal law, the United Kingdom has proceeded along a different path. The GMC, whose powers derive from the Medical Acts, and which is responsible to the Privy Council, has enforced professional standards on the basis of guidance rather than through a codified system.

The views of the medical profession on matters of medical ethics are formulated through resolutions of the Annual Representative Meeting (ARM) of the BMA. The ARM consists of representatives from all branches of the profession throughout the country, thus expressing the views of the profession on medical ethics. This Handbook includes some notes of guidance from the GMC, and the latter's advice on professional conduct makes reference to guidance covered by this publication.

Relationships between doctors and individuals

1 Forms of medical relationship

Introduction

1.1 There are three types of professional relationship between a doctor and a member of the public. The attitude of the person, the constraints on the doctor and the form of the relationship varies in each case. It is the duty of the doctor to tell a person with whom he comes into professional contact the nature of the relationship, and in whose interest he (the doctor) is acting.

Therapeutic doctor-patient relationship

1.2 In the first form of contact a person may consult a doctor as a patient. The doctor then acts in the interests of the patient and is responsible to the patient for his actions. Most medical work takes this form. (See also 2.12.)

Medical examiner and research work

1.3 A doctor may act as an impartial medical examiner and report to a third party (Chapter 3), or engage in clinical or other research in his own interest, in the interests of a group of people, or in the interests of the advancement of medical science (Chapter 4). In these circumstances the information gathered by the doctor will be used for purposes other than the clinical care of the patient. Thus the patient may properly wish to limit the information he discloses.
1.4 It would be wrong for a doctor to examine a patient on the basis of a normal therapeutic relationship where this does not exist. If the doctor who normally has a therapeutic relationship with the patient is called upon to act in a different role, the nature of the relationship should be carefully explained to the patient. Similar constraints apply when a patient is involved in a medical research project conducted by his own doctor.

11

Confidentiality

1.5 The nature of professional confidence varies according to the form of consultation or examination but, in each of the three forms of relationship, the doctor is responsible to the patient or person with whom he is in a professional relationship for the security and confidentiality of information given to him.

1.6 A doctor must preserve secrecy on all he knows. There are five exceptions to this general principle:

(1) The patient gives consent.

(2) When it is undesirable on medical grounds to seek a patient's consent, but is in the patient's own interest that confidentiality should be broken.

(3) The doctor's overriding duty to society.

(4) For the purposes of medical research, when approved by a local clinical research ethical committee, or in the case of the National Cancer Registry by the Chairman of the BMA's Central Ethical Committee or his nominee. (See Chapter 4.)

(5) When the information is required by due legal process.

1.7 A doctor must be able to justify his decision to disclose information. When making a decision to breach confidentiality and disclose information concerning a patient the doctor should always remember that he may, at any time, be required to justify his actions.

Consent to disclosure

1.8 The information that a patient gives to a doctor remains the property of the patient, who may authorise the doctor to share this with anyone the patient wishes. The doctor is responsible for limiting the disclosure of medical information to the extent to which consent has been given. Every effort should be made to enable the patient to understand the implications of releasing information, and the extent of the proposed disclosure. Beyond the necessary sharing of information with other persons concerned with the clinical care of the patient (both for any particular episode or, where essential, for the continuing care of the patient), the patient's consent must be obtained before disclosure. This consent is valid only if the patient fully understands the nature and consequences of the disclosure.

1.9 Information shared with other doctors or members of other health professions may be given in the normal form of clinical report. In all other cases it must be presented in the form of a report appropriate to the circumstances.

Exceptional circumstances

1.10 Circumstances do arise which render it undesirable for a patient to be told the full implications of his condition. Whilst a doctor clearly cannot obtain consent to disclose information, he is not prevented from giving relevant information to a relative or other appropriate person having regard to the particular circumstances.

Duty to society

1.11 A doctor, like every other citizen, is a member of society with all the responsibilities this entails. Occasions may arise in which these persuade the doctor that confidential information acquired in the course of a medical consultation must be disclosed. In line with the principles of medical secrecy, wherever possible the doctor should seek to persuade the patient to disclose the information himself or give permission for the doctor to disclose it. Failing this, it will be for the doctor and for his own conscience to decide on his further course of action.

1.12 In the course of their professional career, many doctors will receive requests from the police for access to personal medical information. When considering the balance between the public interest and his duty to the individual patient, a doctor should start from the premise that information given to him by a patient in the course of a professional consultation must be kept secret. There are clearly occasions when the balance of the public interest—where enquiries relate to a very grave crime where the security of the public is at risk—will so outweigh the doctor's duty to an individual patient that his decision will be easy. On other occasions the balance will be finely drawn. A doctor must be aware that if, after the most careful consideration, he decides to transmit information which was given to him in confidence to the police, he may be called upon to justify his action subsequently, either before the General Medical Council or in a court of law.

1.13 Doctors who have difficulty in reaching a decision, having considered the facts presented to them by the police, are advised to discuss such requests with their local BMA liaison officer, the Head Office of the BMA, or their defence body.

The law

1.14 Medical information required by law or statute falls into two categories; that which is required by statutory instrument, and individual cases in which an order is made by a Court of Law.

1.15 Some of the accepted situations and circumstances in which a doctor is required by Act of Parliament to do, or not do, certain things are set out in Chapter 9. Professional discipline is exercised under statute by the General Medical Council, within guidelines issued from time to time.

1.16 In the United Kingdom no privilege attaches to communications between patient and doctor, and a doctor can therefore be directed by a Court to disclose such information. A refusal to comply with such a direction could lead to the doctor being held to be in contempt of Court. When asked by a Court to disclose information without the patient's consent, the doctor should refuse on the grounds of professional confidence and say why he feels that disclosure should not be enforced. The Court would normally take the doctor's statement into consideration but if in spite of this he is ordered to answer the questions, the decision whether to comply or not must be for his own conscience. A decision to refuse, while illegal, is not necessarily unethical (see also 6.6).

The Courts and legal proceedings

1.17 The law relating to the disclosure of medical records for the purposes of litigation in claims based on personal injury or death is now contained in Sections 33 and 34 of the Supreme Court Act 1981. Broadly, these empower the Court to order the disclosure of medical records to:

(a) a person who is an actual or potential litigant;
(b) his legal adviser; or
(c) a medical adviser nominated by him, or
(d) a combination of (b) and (c).

The discretion in deciding which of these methods to use is that of the Court and any doctor who is in doubt as to the most suitable

14

procedure in any given case is strongly advised to consult his medical defence body.

1.18 Doctors who are approached by solicitors for access to records are advised to seek advice from the BMA or their defence body, as the law on this subject is now so complicated.

Storage and access to clinical information

1.19 The doctor must ensure, as far as he can, that all medical information is kept in a secure place.

1.20 The following statements apply to records systems in all disciplines of medical practice, and set out the basic criteria for access to records which include clinical information:

(a) In all medical records, information should be regarded as held for the specific purpose of the continuing care of the patient, and should not be used, without appropriate authorisation by the responsible clinician or the consent of the patient, for any other purpose.

(b) Access to identifiable information held in medical records should be restricted to the author and the person clinically responsible for the patient during the episode for which the data were collected (or their successor) unless specifically authorised by the clinician in the interests of the patient. Access to clinical data of previous episodes of illness should be available to the clinicians currently providing care for the patient. Access to such information should only be allowed, where practicable, with the patient's consent.

(c) An individual should not be indentifiable from data supplied for statistical or research purposes. If follow-up of the individual patient is a necessary part of the research, the patient must have previously given consent. Consent to the release of information for a medical research project must have been obtained from a local ethical committee for clinical research, or in the case of the National Cancer Registry, from the Chairman of the BMA's Central Ethical Committee. (See Chapter 4.)

1.21 In view of his responsibility to ensure that confidentiality is preserved, when a doctor has doubts about the security and confidentiality of his patients' records in any record storage system he should refuse to place clinical information in them.

15

2 The doctor in personal medical care

2.1 A person is free to choose the doctor from whom he wishes to obtain medical advice. Equally a doctor is free to accept or refuse any person as a patient, subject to the constraints of his professional obligations, such as:

(a) In an emergency where a doctor is bound to provide any treatment immediately necessary and to ensure that arrangements are made for any necessary further treatment.

(b) In isolated communities where the doctor is the only source of medical advice.

2.2 However, the organisation and rules of Social Security may have the effect of limiting the choice of those participating in the Scheme. In NHS general practice a Family Practitioner Committee has the power to assign a patient to a doctor whether he agrees or not.

2.3 The fundamental principle remains one of free choice.

Overall management and freedom of choice

2.4 It is good medical practice for one doctor to be responsible for the overall management of a patient's illness.

2.5 Occasionally a patient may wish to approach a doctor other than his usual medical practitioner. This occurs particularly when a patient has difficulty in attending his usual practitioner because his work area is some distance from home. If the patient is not under active treatment by his usual practitioner, a doctor is free to accept him as a patient, although the doctor may wish to consult the patient's usual practitioner in accordance with good medical practice. Such consultations must have the consent of the patient.

2.6 If a patient is already under treatment but chooses to consult another doctor, he must accept that normally the doctor will refuse to treat him unless he terminates the previous clinical relationship. If this course is adopted the patient should inform his previous doctor that he is receiving care from another medical practitioner (see also 2.7 below).

2.7 Other than in an emergency, a doctor in whatever form of practice should take positive steps to satisfy himself that a patient who applies for treatment or advice is not already under the active care of another practitioner before he accepts him. If the patient is under active treatment he should be informed of the reasons why his usual medical practitioner should be contacted before medical care is initiated. If the patient does not consent to this procedure, the doctor may refuse to treat him unless the patient is prepared to terminate the previous clinical relationship (see 2.6).

2.8 Having taken account of the principles set out in 2.6 and 2.7, where a doctor agrees to undertake the care of a patient, he must accept the responsibility of continuing care, including the issue of any necessary prescriptions (see also 6.8).

Referral to consultants and specialists

2.9 Referral from a general practitioner to a consultant or specialist has evolved in the patient's interest. The General Medical Council, in its booklet *Professional Conduct and Discipline: Fitness to Practice* (August 1983), has stated:

> "*Acceptance of patients by specialists*
> Although an individual patient is free to seek to consult any doctor, the Council wishes to affirm its view that, in the interests of the generality of patients, a specialist should not usually accept a patient without reference from the patient's general practitioner. If a specialist does decide to accept a patient without such reference, the specialist has the duty immediately to inform the general practitioner of his findings and recommendation before embarking on treatment, except in emergency, unless the patient expressly withholds consent or has no general practitioner. In such cases the specialist must be responsible for the patient's subsequent care until another doctor has agreed to take over that responsibility.
> In expressing this view the Council recognises and accepts that in some areas of practice specialist and hospital clinics customarily accept patients referred by sources other than their general practitioners. In these circumstances the specialist still has the duty to keep the general practitioner informed."

2.10 A medical practitioner may have special skills: for example, he may use acupuncture or hypnosis as part of his treatment of cases. The use of these skills in relation to a patient for whom he is not the usual medical practitioner constitutes practice analogous to that of a specialist. If he accepts a patient without reference from a general practitioner (other than in the circumstances set out in paragraph 2.11 below) he must observe the guidance set out in paragraphs 2.7 and 2.8 above.

2.11 A doctor in consultant or specialist practice should not accept a patient without reference from a general practitioner except in the following circumstances:

(*a*) In an emergency.

(*b*) If he is asked for a confirmatory opinion or specialist opinion on a different aspect of the case by the specialist to whom the patient has been properly referred.

(*c*) If reference back to the general practitioner would produce delay seriously detrimental to the patient. The specialist should inform the general practitioner as soon as possible of the action he has taken and the reasons for it.

(*d*) If referred by doctors in the school or other community child services—but only after the general practitioner has been given the opportunity to refer the child himself.

(*e*) If it is for a consultation in venereology.

(*f*) If inquiry indicates that the consultation is for a refraction examination only.

(*g*) If a patient is formally referred by a physician from outside the United Kingdom.

(*h*) If the patient is seeking contraceptive advice and treatment and is unwilling to consult her own general practitioner about contraception, or she states that her own general practitioner does not provide contraceptive services. At the time the advice and treatment is sought it should be explained to the patient that it is in her own best interests that her general practitioner be informed that contraception has been prescribed and of any medical condition discovered which requires investigation or treatment. Every attempt should be made to obtain permission to contact the general practitioner prior to prescription or fitting of a contraceptive device. This is particularly important if the patient is at the same time under the active clinical care of her own general practitioner or that of another doctor.

(*i*) If the patient is seeking therapeutic abortion and is unwilling to consult her own general practitioner or, having done so, is unable to secure his agreement to refer her to another doctor. It should be explained to the patient that it is in her own best interest that her general practitioner be informed of the treatment or advice given. Every attempt should be made to obtain the permission of the patient for this.

Consent to treatment

2.12 The patient's trust that his consent to treatment will not be misused is an essential part of his relationship with his doctor. For a doctor even to touch a patient without consent may constitute an assault.

2.13 Consent is only valid when freely given by a patient who understands the nature and consequences of what is proposed.

2.14 Assumed consent or consent obtained by undue influence is valueless (see also 4.9). It is particularly important that consent should be free of any form of pressure or coercion, and especially where treatment is offered to patients such as those serving in the Armed Forces or other type of employment which limit freedom of action of the individual. No influence should be exerted through any special relationship between a doctor and the person whose consent is sought.

2.15 Doctors offer advice but it is the patient who decides whether or not to accept the advice. The necessary degree of understanding of what is proposed depends on the patient's education and intelligence and the seriousness and urgency of the condition being investigated or treated. The onus is always on the doctor carrying out the procedure to see that an adequate explanation is given.

Minors

2.16 Section 8(1) of the *Family Law Reform Act 1969* states that "the consent of a minor who has attained the age of sixteen years to any surgical, medical or dental treatment which, in the absence of consent, would constitute a trespass to his person shall be as effective as it would be if he were of full age: and where a minor has by virtue of this section given an effective consent to any treatment, it shall not be necessary to obtain any consent for it from his parent or guardian". Section 8(3) says "nothing in this section shall be construed as making ineffective any consent which would have been effective if this section had not been enacted". This sub-section arises from uncertainty as to the common law position before the passing of the Act.

2.17 A common problem is that of a patient under the age of 16 who requires treatment when no parent or guardian is available. Emergencies should not wait for consent and there can be little doubt that a court, having regard to parents' duty to provide medical care for their child, will uphold the doctor's action in providing such care as might reasonably anticipate the parents' consent. Where there is difficulty in contacting the parents, the doctor must assess the urgency of the need for treatment before embarking on any procedure.

Minors and contraception

2.18 Opinions have been expressed that doctors providing contraception, even with the parents' consent, for minors under the age of 16 might be aiding and abetting the offence of unlawful sexual intercourse. Legal advice is that, if a doctor acts in good faith in protecting the girl against the potentially harmful effects of intercourse, he would not be acting unlawfully.

2.19 Where a girl under the age of 16 requests contraception but refuses to allow her parents to be informed, the question of the validity of the girl's consent is raised. It appears that Section 8(3) of the *Family Law Reform Act 1969* would consider such consent valid in certain cases (see 2.16).

2.20 When faced with this problem a doctor should take the following steps:

> (*a*) Attempt to convince the girl of the advisability of involving her parents in this decision. This should be part of the counselling extended over a number of interviews, where appropriate. In many cases the doctor will gain consent to involve the parents.
>
> (*b*) If he is unsuccessful, the doctor must then decide whether the girl has the mental maturity to understand the possible consequences of her action. If she has not, then her consent is not informed and so invalid.
>
> (*c*) If he is satisfied that she can consent, he makes a clinical decision as to whether the provision of contraception is in the best interests of the patient. A decision not to prescribe does not absolve him from keeping the interview confidential.

Incapacity to consent

2.21 Except when a guardian has been appointed, no individual or office holder has legal authority to consent to treatment being given to an adult who is mentally incapable of making a decision. The fact that a patient has been admitted to hospital under a section of the relevant *Mental Health Act,* or is an informal patient in a mental hospital does not necessarily indicate his ability to give or to withhold consent. The patient's right to give or withhold consent to treatment for a physical condition is not lessened by the fact of his being admitted under such an Act. What must be considered is whether the patient is able to appreciate the reasons for the nature of, and the possible complications of the proposed treatment, and what would happen if the proposed treatment were withheld.

Consent to operations on reproductive organs

2.22 The custom of obtaining the consent of the patient's spouse to operations on the reproductive organs is one of courtesy not of legal necessity. Nevertheless, because the patient's partner may properly hold that he or she has an interest in such an operation, it is good practice to attempt to obtain consent from both partners (see also 9.7 on the consent of both partners to AID). Similar considerations apply to the investigation or treatment of the fetus or embryo, or of the intra-uterine environment, particularly as the fetus is incapable of giving any consent.

Trust

2.23 The General Medical Council has said of the relationship between doctors and their patients:

> "Patients grant doctors privileged access to their homes and confidences. . . . Good medical practice depends upon the maintenance of trust between doctors and patients and their families, and the understanding by both that proper professional relationships will be strictly observed. In this situation doctors must exercise great care and discretion in order not to damage this crucial relationship."

2.24 The relationship between patient and doctor is based on trust. The doctor will be constantly on his guard to be objective in his judgment in the face of the many outside pressures which may be exerted on him. These may be economic, or pressures from relatives, advertising, the media, or from other sources.

2.25 A doctor is entitled to decline to provide any treatment which he believes to be wrong, but there is a distinction between treatment which a doctor believes to be detrimental to a patient's best interests, and treatment to which a doctor has a conscientious objection. A doctor must not allow his decision as to what is in the

21

patient's best interests to be influenced by his own personal beliefs. If a person who is already a doctor's patient requests treatment which that doctor believes to be against the patient's best interests, he should tell the patient and point out that the patient has the right to seek advice elsewhere. If a person who is already a doctor's patient is found by the doctor to need treatment which the doctor cannot provide or take part in because of the doctor's own principles, the doctor must tell the patient and ensure that the patient is referred to alternative medical care (see also 10.3).

Communication

Doctor and patient

2.26 The commonest cause of problems between doctors and patients is failure of communication. Clear communication is of fundamental importance, not only in establishing a clear rapport between the parties but also as an essential part of the diagnostic and therapeutic process. The doctor must choose his words with care, not only to ensure that the patient provides an unambiguous reply to the questions posed during the diagnostic process, but also to ensure that no misunderstanding occurs in giving any information to the patient concerning his condition, the regime of treatment proposed (with side effects explained where appropriate) and also the prognosis. Particular care should be taken to avoid misunderstanding if technical words are used.

Professional colleagues

2.27 Rapid and clear communication between professional colleagues engaged in the care of a patient is essential. If continuity of care is to be properly maintained, essential information must be available to the physician who becomes responsible for that patient's immediate continuing care. This applies, for example, where a patient under treatment by his medical practitioner moves to another area, or when a patient enters or is discharged from hospital. It is vital that a preliminary discharge letter is sent, which is clearly legible. The doctor from whose immediate care the patient is passing should decide the best means of communication, having regard to the circumstances and the likely delay in receipt of a posted letter. The use of abbreviations should be avoided wherever possible, as they may lead to misunderstanding.

2.28 Letters of referral to a colleague and requests for specialist diagnostic investigations should make reference to any aspects of the patient's history which, though not of immediate relevance to the subject of referral, might be of importance in any action by the specialist.

2.29 Failure to communicate essential information could be construed as medical negligence in a professional sense, since it departs from one of the most important tenets of good medical practice.

Doctors in specialised communities

2.30 Doctors who serve specialised communities may face additional ethical problems. The peculiar nature of the environment may modify the balance between the doctor's duty of professional confidence to his patient, and the overriding needs of the community. These groups include:

Prison medical officers
Armed Forces medical officers
Ships' surgeons
Expedition doctors

Prison medical officers

2.31 A prisoner cannot usually choose his doctor. Apart from this single restriction a prisoner has a right to the same medical attention as any other member of society, and a prison medical officer's responsibility to, and professional relationship with, his patients is the same as that of any doctor working outside prison. He will have particular regard to the advice given in paragraphs 2.12–2.15 on consent to treatment (see also 4.9 and 6.11–6.22).

Armed Forces medical officers

2.32 A doctor in the Armed Forces has to obey any lawful command that is given to him. Disobedience is an offence punishable by court martial. It is obvious that the command may conflict with his ethical responsibilities. In all three services a serving doctor is responsible for his professional actions to the same extent as a civilian medical practitioner and he is expected to work within the same ethical

23

constraints as the rest of the profession. The ethical freedom of serving medical officers is guarded by the medical Directors General. They have accepted that they must ensure that no medical officer can be required to treat a patient in accordance with a given policy when the doctor believes that the treatment is not in that individual's best interests.

2.33 A patient who consults a doctor in the services should be aware that the duty of the doctor to keep secret the information given to him is importantly modified. When a person joins the services he tacitly consents to give up some of the freedoms of civilian life. One of these is strict confidentiality, because there are times when a medical officer is required to discuss cases with his commanding officer in the interests of the unit as a whole.

2.34 When a serviceman takes his family on an accompanied posting, the health of the family may affect both the serviceman and the unit. The special relationship between the serviceman, his medical officer, and the commanding officer does not extend to the family. So the medical officer may discuss the implications but not the clinical details.

2.35 The ethical standards set out in Chapter 6 relating to interrogation and punishment apply both to serving medical officers and to civilian practitioners.

Ships' surgeons

2.36 Medical officers employed in the Merchant Navy work in an environment that is similar in one respect to that of Armed Forces doctors. The community may be put in danger if the captain of a ship is unaware that a member of the crew is incapable of carrying out his duties, or that a passenger is so ill as to constitute a risk to other people on board.

2.37 The medical officer's decision in these circumstances is a negative one. Unless he decides that the damage to his patient will be out of proportion to the risk of giving information obtained from his work to the captain, the doctor should feel able to discuss cases in outline if he believes that there is a risk to others in the community.

Expedition doctors

2.38 The relationships between the members of an expedition, the medical officer, and the expedition leader are similar to those on a ship.

3 The doctor as an impartial expert

3.1 The second form of contact occurs when a person is examined by a doctor who reports the outcome of his examination to a third party.

3.2 Consent to an examination carried out in these circumstances is essential unless the examination is ordered under statutory authority (Chapter 9), and even then a doctor may refuse to examine a person against his will. The person's lack of collaboration is then a matter between him and the statutory authority.

3.3 A person may properly wish to limit the information he discloses to a doctor who will report to a third party. Police surgeons, occupational physicians, and doctors carrying out life assurance and other examinations should make sure that the person understands the doctor's role before the examination starts.

3.4 Should the person being examined already be a patient of the doctor, the doctor must ensure that he distinguishes between his two roles. Since he is acting as an expert examiner reporting on the objective findings of his examination, he must not allow information gathered in his "therapeutic role" to form the basis of his report as an expert.

Community medicine

3.5 Community medicine is that medical specialty which deals with populations or groups rather than with individual patients. In the context of a national system of health care it comprises those doctors who try to measure the needs of the population, both sick and well, who plan and administer services to meet those needs and those who are engaged in research and teaching in the field.

3.6 Community physicians face ethical problems of a different nature. They fall into three general categories: (1) those affecting the individual patient and the community; (2) those affecting the doctor's own personal views and standards; and (3) those affecting the doctor's relationships with his colleagues.

The individual and the community

3.7 While the community physician will normally find himself advising a health authority on decisions affecting the needs of one

25

group of society as opposed to another, he may also from time to time be called upon to advise the authority on matters relating to an individual. In these circumstances he may have to balance the rights of the individual against those of society as a whole.

Provision of services contrary to individual ethical beliefs

3.8 Services contrary to the beliefs and ethical standards of some doctors have been introduced by legislation. For example, abortion and contraception for the unmarried may present special problems to doctors appointed to advise authorities on the provision of services.

3.9 The community physician may find himself giving advice to a Health Authority which serves people with many different ethical views. He may be unable to ascertain the wishes of them all and therefore unable to decide whether he should support the provision of a service with which he personally disagrees, or whether it is enough to state his own view and then in his executive capacity implement the authority's decision. The community physician has a duty to assess the need as accurately as possible and to be aware of the dangers inherent in the method of assessment. He must also keep economic factors in mind and if resources need to be allocated for more urgent things he should say so. If a community physician is satisfied that there is a case for the introduction of a service, it would be unrealistic and inappropriate for him to oppose it, even though he disagrees with it on personal ethical grounds. He has a moral duty, however, to continue to declare his own ethical position and is entitled to persuade others that it is the most appropriate one.

Intra-professional relations

3.10 Relations with clinical colleagues are well illustrated by consideration of medical recommendations for re-housing. Local Authority councillors may argue that they cannot effectively deal with applications for re-housing without a detailed understanding of the medical background. The ethical situation of the community physician is complex. He has no clinical relationship with the patient and may feel compelled to recommend a course of action contrary to that requested by the patient. The clinician may, with the consent of the patient, reveal medical facts to the community physician. The community physician is ethically accountable for what he does with this information. In other circumstances,

26

however, the clinician may, with the patient's consent, complete a form from which conclusions can be drawn where wider non-medical circulation is intended. When such a document is forwarded to the community physician, his task is to formulate the relevant conclusions for the organisation to which it is directed and not to assume the clinician's responsibility for the confidentiality of any information so conveyed.

Occupational medicine

3.11 The position of the occupational physician presents particular problems. He is appointed by his company and is responsible for the occupational health of all employed therein, individually and collectively. He deals constantly with other doctors' patients. These considerations in no way alter the doctor/patient relationship. The fact that he is a salaried employee of the company gives no other employee of that company any right of access to medical records or to the details of examination findings. With the patient's consent the employer may be advised of information relating to a specific matter, the significance of which the patient clearly understands.

3.12 The ethical position of the occupational physician will be clearly defined if the need to undergo medical examinations required by statute or company policy is referred to in the contracts of the employees affected. The nature of the examination and the need for disclosure of the significance of the findings should be set out in the contract or in the corresponding reference documents.

3.13 If an employer explicitly or implicitly invites members of his staff to consult the occupational physician the latter must still regard such consultations as confidential. *The Health and Safety at Work Act 1974* has had a substantial effect upon the involvement of the occupational physician with a larger percentage of the population. Nevertheless, the principles which follow must still be applied when the occupational physician has to concern himself with an individual patient.

Intra-professional relations

3.14 The occupational physician should treat patients only in co-operation with the patient's general practitioner except in an emergency. This applies also to the use of any special facilities or staff which he may have. Before telling the general practitioner of

27

any findings or treatment, he should obtain the person's consent to do so.

3.15 If the occupational physician believes that the worker should consult his general practitioner, he should urge him to do so.

3.16 The occupational physician should refer a patient directly to hospital only in consultation or in agreement with the general practitioner.

3.17 The occupational physician does not usually have to confirm that absence from work is due to sickness. If the occupational physician proposes to examine a worker who is or has been absent for health reasons, he should inform the general practitioner on matters of substance, so that the general practitioner can contribute to the final opinion to be expressed by the occupational physician.

3.18 The occupational physician should not give opinions as to liability in accidents at work or individual diseases without the consent of the parties concerned, except when legally required to do so.

3.19 Occupational physicians should not influence—or appear to influence—any worker in his choice of general practitioner.

Employment medical advisers and occupational physicians

3.20 Many of the conflicts of interest in occupational medicine are similar to those already outlined. In particular, statutory and other periodic medical examinations may affect continued employment in a particular job. The patient must be reminded of the doctor's role as the agent of a third party. Airline pilots, workers in the atomic energy industry, and medical staff developing allergies to drugs are examples of the difficult cases which have to be tackled. So too are employees whose sickness absence record is substantial. In these cases an industrial tribunal will have to be satisfied that the doctor has acted equitably. While the employer has no right to clinical detail of sickness or injury, the doctor he employs can be reasonably expected to interpret those details in terms of

—the likely date of return to work, if at all;
—the likely disability of the patient at that time;
—the term of the disability.

3.21 The Medical Advisory Committee of the Health and Safety Executive is reviewing the need for periodic statutory investigations in various industries and processes (see also 9.8). The employee has rights analogous to the patient being examined by a police doctor, in that he may refuse to be examined, but must bear the consequences of that refusal.

3.22 Individual clinical findings are confidential, though their significance may be conveyed to a third party. Thus, while an individual reading of a laboratory result may not be published, it may be proper to disclose that an individual or a group show a significant degree of exposure to a potentially toxic hazard.

Police surgeons

3.23 A police surgeon may not only have to examine patients on behalf of the police, but also to examine and treat ill patients in custody. The doctor should be clear where his responsibilities lie. It would be improper for him to disregard the ordinary guidelines for confidentiality (Chapter 1) when he is treating a detained person as a patient (see also 6.21–6.22).

Examination

3.24 The police surgeon should identify himself to the person to be examined and explain the purpose of the examination, and of any specimen which may be requested. The person in custody is not obliged to submit to medical examination or treatment, or to provide specimens for forensic examination. In the absence of consent, therefore, any treatment or attempt to obtain specimens would constitute an assault.

3.25 Where the consent of the person in custody has been obtained, the examination should, if possible, be witnessed by a third party. A police officer may be present but should not be within earshot. In the case of a woman in custody, a policewoman or other female should be present. If a solicitor wishes to be present during the examination, the consent of the accused should be obtained.

Fitness for custody and observation

3.26 The information obtained on examination is confidential and only sufficient detail should be given to the police to enable them to take proper care of the individual. In the cases of serious illnesses some information may be given, but not if the illness is the result of the patients indiscretion, eg venereal disease. Information obtained as a result of *observation* where consent to examination has been

29

refused may not be revealed without the consent of the accused, except on the direction of a court.

Minors

3.27 Relatives may be present at the examination of a person under the age of 16 if they request it. If no relatives are available a minor may have to be placed under legal guardianship in order that consent may be obtained (see also 2.16).

Unconscious patient

3.28 Examination and procedures to ensure the life of a person in custody may be carried out without consent if the person is unconscious. Specimens may be taken for biochemical investigations, ie diagnostic purposes, but the results of tests must not be used for forensic purposes without the subsequent consent of the patient. If the individual is under 16 a parent or guardian can give consent to these procedures.

4 Research in human subjects

4.1 The third form of contact with doctors occurs in the field of research. The law lays down a minimum code in matters of professional negligence and the doctrine of assault, but this is not enough. Most patients trust their doctors and will seriously consider any proposal in connection with research. For practical purposes, the doctor concerned carries a moral responsibility for the investigations that are, or are not, proposed to his patient or volunteer. As full an explanation as possible must be given (see 2.26).

4.2 .Medical advances have always depended upon the public's confidence in those who carry out investigations on human subjects. This confidence will be maintained only if the public believes that such investigations are submitted to rigorous ethical scrutiny and self-discipline. It is unethical to conduct research which is badly planned or poorly executed.

4.3 Codes, regulations and laws help to keep standards of ethical behaviour high, but volunteers and patients are best protected by ethical conduct. The subjects' interests must come first. The general rules governing the conduct of this type of research are contained in the Declaration of Helsinki, which is reproduced in full in the Chapter on Ethical Codes and Statements.

Controlled clinical trials

4.4 Controlled trials are useful in deciding the value of a particular type of therapy when comparable groups of subjects are available. The comparison may be with a procedure previously generally accepted as valuable, or with a placebo, or both. Consent must be obtained from the individual subjects: when obtained by a member of the investigating team, it should be obtained before randomisation if that is part of the method.

4.5 A Code of Practice for Assessment of Licensed Medicines in General Practice has been published by the Association of British Pharmaceutical Industries. In future every protocol sent to a doctor will be accompanied by a copy of the ABPI Code.

4.6 Because of the ethical problems which may arise, controlled clinical trials should always be approved and supervised by a properly constituted ethical committee. The BMA has published a model constitution for local ethical committees, which has received support from the representative organisations of all branches of the medical profession. Adequate background information must be provided to any ethical committee to allow the scientific merit of the proposal to be judged as well as the ethics.

4.7 Any doctor remains free to remove a patient under his care from such a trial, or to give additional treatment at any time if he feels it to be in the patient's best interest. Similarly, any patient is free to withdraw.

Research on children

4.8 Investigators who plan projects which require research on children should pay attention to the following points:

(a) The investigator must ask himself if the project can only be carried out with the use of children.

(b) The project should be submitted to the local ethical committee for clinical research for approval. The investigator should indicate the method he will use to obtain consent ie, from the parents and/or the general practitioner, or consultant in charge of the case.

31

(c) For pregnant women, infants, and children under 10 years of age the requirements for informed consent should be particularly stringent. Parents should be aware of their right to withdraw consent at any time if reflection or experience gives them cause for concern. Unless there are very compelling reasons for not doing so, a brief written statement about the nature and purpose of the project, which can be incorporated in the consent form, should be prepared, and a copy retained by the parents.

Research on prisoners

4.9 Consent obtained by undue influence is valueless. A prisoner might expect benefits from agreeing to participate in a research procedure or controlled trial, even if these had not been offered. It is, therefore, unethical to carry out a research procedure on a prisoner that is of no direct benefit to the affected individual.

Research in occupational medicine

4.10 A doctor in occupational medicine may be called upon to undertake research upon workers in a particular industry for the purpose of statutory investigations (see also 9.8).

Clinical trials of new drugs

4.11 New drugs are assessed at various stages in their development by the Committee on Safety of Medicines (CSM). Hospital doctors and general practitioners may be asked to take part in a clinical trial. They will not be acting unethically if they agree to do so provided they are certain that the trial is necessary and that it will be well organised and executed (see also 2.24).

4.12 The standard protocol for the introduction of a new drug has a number of stages. Once the drug has been synthesised and preliminary investigations suggest that it has pharmaceutical activity, a programme of chemical, pharmaceutical, and animal investigations is started. Data on these investigations, as well as controlled human pharmacological studies, are submitted to the CSM in an application for permission to undertake clinical trials (the *Clinical Trials Submission*).

4.13 If the CSM is satisfied with the data, permission is granted for a limited number—usually three or four—of controlled studies in patients. After analysing the results, together with any other pre-clinical investigations, the CSM allows further clinical trials with more patients.

4.14 Finally, a submission containing all the data is put to the CSM for permission to market the drug (the *Marketing or Product Licence Submission*). From synthesis to marketing rarely takes less than four years. Various types of clinical trials are undertaken in hospitals and in general practice during the earlier stages and when a drug is marketed. General practice studies are often the final step before a marketing submission is made, and more are usually performed when the drug is freely available. These studies are carried out not only to identify the drug's main indications, but also other factors such as efficacy, patient compliance and adverse reactions.

Relationships between doctors and groups

5 The doctor and other groups in society

Social change and multidisciplinary care

5.1 The doctor, traditionally a person of authority, now has his opinions questioned by individuals and groups with increased medical knowledge, with the result that the ethical implications of his actions are under scrutiny as never before.

5.2 Conflict between non-medical staff and their employers may disrupt the medical care of sick people. The doctor is not under any obligation to take new patients under his care (but see 2.1), and should not so so unless he is satisfied that he can treat them properly. He must look after the patients already under his care as well as possible in the circumstances, unwillingly accepting that the actions of others may impede him. If, however, a doctor believes that he cannot look after a patient safely then he should tell his patient and try to arrange for alternative medical care.

5.3 Another change of attitude with ethical implications concerns claims by non-medically qualified people, that doctors should not have sole authority over diagnosis, referral, treatment, the granting of access to resources, and rehabilitation. This development has deep significance for patients, for all the health professions, and for the health services.

Paramedical professions and professions supplementary to medicine

5.4 The professions must find ways of protecting the right of the individual to confidential communication with any professional person he chooses. A doctor may trust the person to whom he discloses information either because he knows him personally, or because his profession is subject to similar ethical standards with adequate sanctions, as are nurses and members of the professions supplementary to medicine, by virtue of their registration with the General Nursing Council and the Council for Professions Supplementary to Medicine.

5.5 When working with a member of one of the other professions, a doctor's duty is to reveal only sufficient information about a patient for the patient's clinical care. The doctor remains responsible to the patient for the confidentiality of that information after he has given it. In deciding whether or not, or how much information to disclose, the doctor must also consider the recipient's standing within his profession.

5.6 The doctor must not have a financial relationship with other practitioners in a professional relationship with the same patient. Such a relationship, particularly if fees are shared, may influence or appear to influence the medical practitioner's treatment of his patients.

Improper delegation of medical duties

5.7 In its booklet *Professional Conduct and Discipline: Fitness to Practise* (August 1983), the General Medical Council stated:

"The Council recognises and welcomes the growing contribution made to health care by nurses and other persons who have been trained to perform specialised functions, and it has no desire either to restrain the delegation to such persons of treatment or procedures falling within the proper scope of their skills or to hamper the training of medical and other health students. But a doctor who delegates treatment or other procedures must be satisfied that the person to whom they are delegated is competent to carry them out. It is also important that the doctor should retain ultimate responsibility for the management of his patients because only the doctor has received the necessary training to undertake this responsibility.

For these reasons a doctor who improperly delegates to a person who is not a registered medical practitioner functions requiring the knowledge and skill of a medical practitioner is liable to disciplinary proceedings. Accordingly the Council has in the past proceeded against those doctors who employed assistants who were not medically qualified to conduct their practices. It has also proceeded against doctors who by signing certificates or prescriptions or in other ways have enabled persons who were not registered medical practitioners to treat patients as though they were so registered." (See also 8.29.)

36

Communication

5.8 The practice of medicine necessitates frequent communication with other professions. This is increasingly the case and the physician has at all time a "duty of clarity". Whether engaged in discussion in the multidisciplinary forum, telephoning instructions to a ward, or writing a prescription or other therapeutic note, the doctor should aim to eliminate ambiguity, doubt or illegibility. Clear messages diminish the possibility of mistakes and harm to patients.

Health professions and the team concept

5.9 As the person who is legally responsible for the treatment and management of a patient and the consequences of decisions in this connection it is logical that the doctor, as the only one who holds this responsibility, should be the director of the medical team. In doing so he will, of course, recognise individuals' professional competences and seek, as appropriate, help and skills from other members of the team, appreciating that some of these skills are properly exercised without reference to the doctor. These considerations must be taken into account in reading the following paragraphs concerning the health professions and the professions supplementary to medicine. (See also 2.27–2.29.)

Nurses and midwives

5.10 Nurses and midwives belong to professions which have their own standards and particular expertise.

5.11 The Royal College of Nursing (RCN) set up a Working Party in 1983 to review the RCN's published documents on a series of issues, including ethical matters. In the case of medical treatment nurses are under an obligation to carry out a doctor's instructions, except where they have a good reason to believe that harm will be caused to the patient by so doing. In cases in which nurses' continuous contact with the patient has given them a different insight into the patient's medical needs, they are under a moral obligation to communicate this to the doctor in charge of the case.

5.12 A nurse may on occasion be more aware of the needs of a patient than a doctor, and the relationship between nurses and doctors should be based upon respect for each other's area of expertise within the framework of the doctor's ultimate responsibility.

5.13 It must be reiterated that it is unethical for a doctor to delegate work unless he has satisfied himself of the competence of the person concerned. The competence of a nurse may vary considerably according to the type of training undertaken, and the experience gained during training.

5.14 Under the law, a trained and registered midwife is permitted to deliver total care on her own responsibility to a woman and her baby during the antenatal, intranatal, postnatal and neonatal periods provided that complications are neither present nor arise. Most practising midwives work within the maternity services team in the hospitals, general practitioner units, and in the community, but an increasing number are self-employed.

5.15 A midwife is required to call in a registered medical practitioner in accordance with the Nurses, Midwives and Health Visitors Rules (NM & HV) 1983 if complications are present or arise at any time. In such cases she is required to carry out the instructions of the doctor in attendance.

5.16 The NM and HV Rules 1983 require a midwife to ensure that before undertaking treatment outside her province or for which she has not previously been trained, she receives the necessary training and considers herself to be competent. Therefore if a doctor wishes to delegate responsibilities to a midwife which are outside her normal sphere of practice she will expect to receive the necessary instruction.

Professions supplementary to medicine

5.17 At the moment, the professions supplementary to medicine include: chiropodists, dietitians, medical laboratory scientific officers (MLSOs) (formerly laboratory technicians who do not treat patients), occupational therapists, orthoptists, physiotherapists, radiographers and remedial gymnasts. Under the *Professions Supplementary to Medicine Act 1960*, each of the professions has a Board and a disciplinary committee. There is a co-ordinating council for the professions supplementary to medicine. Within the NHS the members of these professions, with the exception of chiropodists, treat only those patients referred by registered medical practioners.

5.18 The Disciplinary Statement of each Board underlines the maintenance of high standards of professional conduct. A doctor should make sure that the people to whom he refers patients are registered, or in approved training in their profession, that he refers patients properly to them and retains final authority for the continuation or otherwise of the therapy.

5.19 Information given to a doctor by another professional must be treated as confidential. But co-operation between doctors and other professionals must be based on adequate knowledge.

5.20 While not hampering the undergraduate and postgraduate training of medical and other health care students, the medical practitioner can only delegate treatment and other procedures to a person reasonably believed to be competent to carry them out, and must retain ultimate responsibility for the patient's overall management because only the doctor in clinical charge has received the necessary training to undertake this responsibility.

Pharmacists

5.21 Retail pharmacists have always given informal advice to patients. In rural dispensing practices general practitioners undertake much of the work usually done by a pharmacist. It would be unethical for a doctor to ask a pharmacist to undertake work beyond his competence, but he should recognise the pharmacist's special knowledge of drugs and of their side effects and interactions.

5.22 Collusion between doctors and pharmacists for financial gain is reprehensible. A doctor should not arrange a commission from a pharmacist, nor should he hold a financial interest in any pharmacy in the area of his practice. Professional cards should not be handed to pharmacists for distribution. It is undesirable that messages for a doctor be received or left at pharmacies.

5.23 The Pharmaceutical Society has said that a pharmacist should not recommend a doctor or medical practice unless asked to do so. A pharmacist should have no financial interest in the professional work of any doctor, or give people the impression that he has.

Pharmaceutical industry

5.24 There are many aspects of the Association of British Pharmaceutical Industry's Code of Practice which affect doctors in their practice. The Code is reproduced in the front of the Data Sheet Compendium. Particular attention, however, is drawn to the following section of the Code:

"Gifts and Inducements

17.1 Subject to clause 17.2 no gift or financial inducement shall be offered or given to members of the medical profession for purposes of sales promotion.

17.2 Gifts in the form of articles designed as promotional aids, whether related to a particular product or of general utility, may be distributed to members of the medical and allied professions provided the gift is inexpensive and relevant to the practice of medicine or pharmacy."

Osteopathy

5.25 Modern osteopathy maintains that it augments more conventional medicine with a number of diagnostic and therapeutic techniques based on the premise that much symptomatology of musculoskeletal origin is caused by potentially reversible dysfunction which may be more effectively treated by physical measures such as manipulation, rather than the pharmacological or surgical remedies appropriate to pathological processes. Manipulation and osteopathy are not synonymous. The former represents a manual treatment that has been widely employed for fractures, dislocations, joint adhesions, hernia, or abnormal intra-uterine presentation of the fetus, no less than in spinal disorders. Referral by a doctor to a medically qualified osteopath differs in no way from a referral to any other doctor. However, in the case of a non-medically qualified osteopath, referral to or association with these practitioners by doctors is covered by the principles laid down in GMC advice (see 5.7).

Ministers of religion

5.26 Active collaboration between the medical profession and the clergy can be of great value. A spiritual adviser, of any faith, can be in a good position to help the patient. Patients' spiritual needs vary greatly and their wishes must be of paramount importance. Spiritual advisers who work in hospitals gain special experience in dealing with health professionals. The patient's own spiritual adviser has special knowledge of his family and social background from which the doctor can benefit, especially for long stay patients, in cases of terminal illness, and of bereavement.

Social workers

5.27 Social workers, like some other groups, have evolved no effective sanctions to safeguard confidentiality, and there is currently no compulsion on social workers to register with a disciplinary body. The British Association of Social Workers has an ethical code, and is moving towards registration and the setting up of a disciplinary council.

5.28 Confidentiality presents little real difficulty in working relations between doctors and social workers, provided that there is personal confidence between the professionals concerned. However, as the BASW ethical code is not supported by sanctions of the nature exercised by the GMC, GNC or the Council for Professions Supplementary to Medicine, the doctor must bear in mind that he has responsibility for any disclosures he makes.

6 The doctor and the state

6.1 Article 25(i) of the United Nations Declaration of Human Rights refers to the basic right of an individual to the provision of minimum standards of health care. This, and the World Medical Association Declarations, are attempts to develop supra-national principles out of "natural" laws. Article 25(i) has now been overtaken by Article 12 of the United Nations Covenant on Economic, Social and Cultural Rights. This came into force on 3 January 1976 and has been ratified or is adhered to, by over 50 nations. Unlike the older Declaration, this covenant is legally binding on those nations and is of the nature of positive as opposed to natural law. Most countries have additional positive legislation which to a greater or lesser extent provides for and regulates the delivery of health care.

6.2 International agreements and declarations may be global or applicable to a smaller group of countries. Some international ethical declarations and codes are set out in the Chapter on Ethical Codes and Statements. The Council of Europe is active through the work of the Human Rights Commission at Strasbourg. The European Convention of Human Rights under which the Commission works allows the examination of cases brought by a Member country. The judgments made by the Commission have had considerable influence on the states in question and on doctors working within those states.

The European states and the EEC

6.3 The Directives relating to the free movement of doctors in the EEC impose on a doctor who migrates the duty to conform to the ethical code of the host country. There are some aspects of medical ethics which are not absolutely identical in the countries of the EEC, and the UK style of practice is by by means universal. Within the European Community the "Continental" legal system is codified and common law has much less significance. But in interpreting the law no one can escape the clear intent of the law as outlined in the preamble to the legislation.

6.4 Other EEC countries may regulate areas of medical practice not normally the concern of the General Medical Council, such as the conditions of contract between a doctor and a hospital or the conditions under which doctors may form a group.

6.5 A notable exception to the other six members of the original Community is the Netherlands, where there is no detailed legal code. The law gives the doctor the duty to conduct himself so as to retain the confidence of his patients, to ensure his professional competence, and to observe professional secrecy except where the law provides for disclosure.

6.6 The very rigid application of the principles of confidentiality, or secrecy, is a marked feature of all the ethical systems in the six countries of the original EEC. Whereas a UK doctor may refuse to disclose information about his patients only at the discretion of the court (see 1.16), in the original EEC countries medical secrecy is firmly protected by law. The UK doctors are regarded by their European colleagues as having gone a long way towards abandoning the "absolute secrecy" which they defend. Indeed to breach confidentiality is a criminal offence in some countries; this shows the importance attached to it. There exists in all countries certain derogations from this principle of absolute secrecy but codes which superficially appear similar may have significant differences. For example, the Belgian code does not permit the doctor to be released from his duty to safeguard secrecy even when the patient has expressly given his permission. Other principles upon which the European codes are based include:

6.7 In relation to the general principles underlying medical practice:

(*a*) Respect for life.

(*b*) Equality of patients regardless of religion, race or reputation.

(*c*) The obligation to provide emergency care and to ensure the continuity of care.

(*d*) Regard for the independence of the profession.

(*e*) Respect for the dignity of the profession which must not be undermined.

(*f*) The prohibition of all commercial practices and all activity incompatible with the dignity of the profession.

(*g*) Professional secrecy.

6.8 In relation to social security systems:

(*a*) Free choice of doctor by the patient.

(*b*) Freedom of the doctor to prescribe.

(*c*) Direct negotiations between doctor and patient concerning fees.

(*d*) Direct payment of fees by the patient to the doctor.

6.9 The Standing Committee of Doctors in the EEC, founded in 1959, which represents the medical profession within the European Community, has among its subcommittees one dealing with ethics and one dealing with social security. Among the charters prepared and endorsed by the Committee is that of Nuremburg (1970) dealing with the practice of medicine in the Community, which delineates the fundamental rights of patients and doctors (reproduced in the Chapter on Ethical Codes and Statements), and a declaration on Health Care Costs.

6.10 The European Union of General Practitioners (UEMO) has been particularly concerned with the safeguarding of confidentiality, especially in relation to the use of data banks, and has drawn up a list of principles to be observed when medical information is stored in this way (reproduced in the Chapter on Ethical Codes and Statements).

Torture and punishment

6.11 In no circumstances may a doctor do anything to weaken the physical or mental resistance of a human being, except for strictly therapeutic indications in the clinical interest of the patient.

6.12 Beyond the Declaration of Tokyo on Torture and Other Cruel, Inhuman or Degrading Treatment and the International Code of Medical Ethics (both reproduced in the Chapter on Ethical Codes and Statements) a doctor has a special duty to individuals which, in this matter, transcends national interest and security. Doctors having knowledge of any activities covered by the Declaration of Tokyo have a positive obligation to make those activities publicly known.

Torture

6.13 Within every human being is knowledge and fear of pain, the fear of helplessness before unrestrained cruelty. Torture, the deliberate infliction of pain by one human being on another, is a special horror.

6.14 The whole medical profession carries a responsibility for refusing to condone, co-operate with, or participate in any form of torture. Expression of this conviction by the whole profession supports individual doctors who refuse to collaborate in torture.

6.15 It is unethical for a doctor to carry out an examination on a person before that person is interrogated under duress or tortured. Even though the doctor takes no part in the interrogation or torture, his examination of the patient prior to interrogation could be interpreted as condoning it.

6.16 Whether or not a doctor should treat the effects of torture depends on whether the patient wants the doctor's help. The doctor himself must be prepared to use all his skills to help a patient, whatever the cause of the injuries. But if the victim of torture prefers to die, the doctor must respect the patient's wishes.

Punishment

6.17 Close confinement and reduction of diet are punishments allowed by the United Nations Standard Minimum Rules for the treatment of prisoners.

6.18 A doctor may state what components a basic diet needs to contain. If confinement and reduction of diet is controlled, and is not calculated to damage health, it is not considered to be a cruel and inhuman punishment.

6.19 If any diet is so restricted that medical monitoring is necessary it is unhuman, and no doctor should be associated with it. If a doctor is asked to examine a prisoner who is subject to close confinement or reduction of diet, the doctor must decide whether the procedure is excessive and dangerous to the prisoner's health. If so, the doctor should make a written report and then refuse to be further associated with the procedure.

6.20 Corporal punishment and incarceration in a dark cell are both prohibited punishments under the Standard Minimum Rules and a doctor would be acting unethically if he certified a prisoner as fit to undergo either procedure. Attendance at the corporal punishment of a prisoner is unethical.

6.21 It is unethical for a doctor to administer a drug to a prisoner for any purpose other than for his clinical care. Individual restraint, in contrast to the restraint imposed by confinement in a prison, may be necessary for violent prisoners who are a threat to other prisoners, their guardians, or themselves. A doctor may give medical advice on individual restraint where the doctor judges that the clinical condition of a prisoner makes restraint necessary.

6.22 The presence of a doctor during the interrogation of a prisoner is unethical (see Declaration of Tokyo, Chapter on Ethical Codes and Statements). Armed Forces doctors may undertake medical monitoring of personnel who have agreed, as an informed voluntary act, to be trained in techniques of resistance to intensive interrogation (see also 2.32–2.35 concerning the role of Armed Forces doctors).

7 The doctor and the media

7.1 Increasing public interest in health matters has brought doctors more and more into contact with the media. It is therefore essential that doctors should be aware of the ethics involved in dealing with the media.

7.2 Those doctors able to comment authoritatively on medical subjects should be prepared to do so in order that the public may be informed. Those doctors able to help the public with information should regard talking to the media as an extension of their medical practice. They must, however, ensure that they observe the basic ethical guidance in relation to advertising (see 8.9 and 8.10).

7.3 A doctor has the responsibility to ensure that when a subject under discussion is controversial within the medical profession, the producer or editor is made aware of that fact.

7.4 It is unacceptable for a doctor publicly to discuss his own ability in a particular field in such a way as to imply that his methods are superior to those of other doctors.

7.5 Where a doctor receives an individual medical enquiry following a report in the media he may acknowledge the enquiry, but should refer the patient to his usual medical practitioner.

Identification of the doctor

7.6 It is acceptable for the doctor's identity to be revealed in the following circumstances:

—when it does not add to his professional stature;
—when it is in the public interest, such as an announcement by a community physician about an outbreak of a communicable disease;
—when he is speaking on behalf of an identifiable section of the profession;
—when using media primarily aimed at doctors.

7.7 A doctor may use his own name in connection with subjects other than medicine.

7.8 When discussing a medical subject in the lay press, or on radio or television, he may be named only if he confines himself to general terms, avoiding discussion of identifiable individual cases.

7.9 Doctors making statements on behalf of known organisations may be named when this is in the public interest. However, a doctor must not exploit the media to promote any organisation in which he has a financial interest (see also 8.25 and 8.26).

Etiquette, professional discipline and the law

8 The doctor in practice

Setting up in practice

8.1 A doctor may set up in general practice by appointment to an NHS practice vacancy, by purchasing the goodwill of an existing private practice, by entering into an established partnership, or by putting up his "Plate". There is an obligation on a doctor not to damage the practice of a colleague, particularly one with whom he has recently been engaged in a professional association.

8.2 A consultant commencing practice in a particular speciality or changing his area of practice should not make any public announcement. He may properly notify his colleagues of his availability for private consultations by sending a sealed letter to those practitioners whom he might normally expect to be interested. He may wish to include his home address and telephone number and the address and telephone number of the main consulting premises where private appointments can be arranged.

8.3 A general practitioner who may need to notify his patients of a change of address, or of surgery hours, may send a sealed circular letter to the patients of the practice. The circular should be addressed to those patients who are on the practice books and are not known to have transferred themselves to another doctor. A suitable notice may be placed inside the waiting room of the surgery. Neither the press nor any other form of public communication should be used for the purpose of making an announcement.

8.4 The principles set out in 8.2 above apply to general practitioners providing expertise in a particular field of medicine (see 2.10 and 2.11).

8.5 The usual format for a letter announcing a change of practice arrangements or change of consultant practice should include only the following information:

    (a) The name of the practitioner.

(b) Medical qualifications (degrees or diplomas).

(c) Title of the main speciality in the case of a consultant who is altering his practice.

(d) Brief details of the new surgery address and consulting hours if a general practitioner is altering his arrangements.

Premises

8.6 The sharing of premises with members of allied professions, including the professions supplementary to medicine, has been discouraged for many years. This attitude is based on the need to prevent any infringement of the principle of free choice by the patient. Advances in clinical medicine have brought changes in the structure of medical practice, and the present trend is towards closer integration of the various disciplines contributing to the patient care.

8.7 There is no objection to a surgery being located in a large building such as an office block, provided the doctor's rooms are entirely self-contained so that the patients do not pass through the premises of other tenants on their way to or from the surgery. Doctors may practise from the same building as members of other health care professions if the professional premises are separate and have separate entrances and addresses. In inner city areas there are particular problems in the provision of premises, but nevertheless the location of surgeries in hotels or in other buildings which are extensively used by the general public for commercial purposes should be avoided, wherever possible.

8.8 The sharing of premises by general practitioners with specialists is acceptable, provided there is no direction of patients, either explicitly or implicitly, which would restrict the patients' potential freedom of choice. This proviso also applies to general practitioners whose premises are part of a health authority's centre, from which members of the professions supplementary to medicine also practise.

Advertising and publicity

8.9 The BMA *Report on Advertising an the Medical Profession* (1974) commenced with the following paragraph:

"The word 'advertising' must be taken in its broadest sense to include all those ways by which a doctor is made publicly known either by himself or others, without objection on his part, in a manner which can fairly be regarded as for the purpose of obtaining patients or promoting his own financial advantage."

8.10 In its booklet *Professional Conduct and Discipline: Fitness to Practise* (August 1983) the General Medical Council states:

"The medical profession in this country has long accepted the tradition that doctors should refrain from self-advertisement. In the Council's opinion advertising is not only incompatible with the principles which should govern relations between members of a profession but could be a source of danger to the public. A doctor successful at achieving publicity may not be the most appropriate doctor for a patient to consult. In extreme cases advertising may raise illusory hopes of a cure.

The publication in any form of matter commending or drawing attention to the professional attainments or services of one or more doctors can raise a question of advertising. This becomes a professional offence if the doctor or doctors concerned have either personally arranged for such publication or have instigated or sanctioned or acquiesced in such publication by others, and have done so for the purpose of obtaining patients or otherwise promoting their own professional advantage or financial benefit."

"Advertising may arise from notices or announcements displayed, circulated or made public by a doctor in connection with his own practice, if such notices or announcements materially exceed the limits customarily observed by the profession in this country."

8.11 The booklet also contains specific guidelines on questions of advertising arising from relationships between doctors and organisations providing clinical, diagnostic, or medical advisory services.

8.12 The question of advertising may also arise in a number of other contexts such as books by doctors, articles or letters or other items written by or about them in newspapers or magazines, and talks or appearances by doctors on broadcasting or television (these subjects are covered in Chapter 7).

Advertisement of nursing homes and institutions

8.13 Advertising in the lay press of nursing homes and kindred institutions, where medical advice or treatment is not provided, is a long-standing and acceptable custom. There is no objection to the practice of institutions professing to provide medical advice or

49

treatment advertising in the medical press, or in other publications primarily intended for the medical profession. Such advertisements may include the names and qualifications of the resident and attending medical officers, but there should be no laudatory statement of the form of treatment given or the address of the consulting rooms or of the hours of a member of the medical staff at which he sees private patients.

8.14 If a doctor has a financial interest involving his possible financial gain in any institution to which he refers a patient it is desirable that he should disclose this fact to the patient.

8.15 Establishments designated as nursing homes, where medical advice and treatment is provided, are covered by the guidelines produce by the General Medical Council (see 8.11).

Location of doctors' premises

Door plates, notice boards and signposts

8.16 It is important that the public should be informed of the location of doctors' premises. In choosing the wording and size of a sign the doctor should consider the following criteria:

(a) A sign or doorplate should be unostentatious in size and form.

(b) A plate should not carry more than the doctor's name, qualifications and, in small letters, his surgery hours.

(c) In an area where a substantial proportion of the community normally uses another language, it is acceptable for the information on the doctor's plate to be repeated in that language.

(d) No notices or signposts should be larger or repeated more frequently than is necessary to indicate to patients the location of the premises.

(e) Notices or signposts should not be used to draw public attention to the services of one practice at the expense of others.

Titles of health centres or group practices

8.17 The GMC booklet *Professional Conduct and Discipline: Fitness to Practise* (August 1983) states:

"In selecting a name for a health centre or a medical centre, or indeed a collective title for a group or partnership it is desirable to avoid a name which could be interpreted as implying that the services provided in that centre or by that partnership have received some official recognition not extended to other local doctors. For this reason terms such as 'Medical Centre' or 'Health Centre' should not be used in a manner which might imply that doctors using the centre or practising in the partnership enjoy some special status in a particular place or area."

8.18 It is the doctor's responsibility to observe these criteria when he works in premises such as health centres provided by a health authority. If a doctor contemplates working, or practising from such premises, he should satisfy himself that they are observed by the responsible authority.

Directories and lists of doctors

8.19 An entry of a doctor's name in a telephone directory should appear in the ordinary small type. The doctor should neither request nor allow any entry in a special typeface, or any description other than higher qualifications or, in the case of a consultant, his speciality.

8.20 Names of all doctors in any area are listed in the telephone directory's yellow pages under "Physicians and Surgeons". The list does not tend to advertise one doctor's availability or skills at the expense of another's, and is acceptable. For the same reason, it is permissible for a doctor's name to be included in a handbook of local information, provided that the list is open to the whole of the profession in the area, that publication of the names is not dependent on the payment of a fee, and that the names are included under a single heading without any indication of specialties.

Canvassing

8.21 Canvassing for the purpose of obtaining patients, whether done directly or through an agent, and association with or employment by persons or organisations which canvass, is unethical.

Certificates and statements

8.22 Doctors are relied upon to issue certificates for a variety of purposes on the assumption that the truth of the certificate can be accepted without question. A doctor must exercise care in issuing certificates and similar documents, and should not include in them statements which he has not taken appropriate steps to verify.

The doctor's signature

8.23 In general terms the doctor should be aware that his signature on a document validates the information or opinion contained in the document. Therefore no doctor should ever sign a document without fully checking the content of the communication which he is signing. Signing routine forms such as those produced by a mechanical haematological counter means only that the doctor is satisfied that the equipment is operating within satisfactory quality control limits. His signature does not validate the information on an individual form, for he has no knowledge of the particular specimen. However, he remains responsible for any opinion or comment that he expresses upon the results.

8.24 If a doctor in civilian practice or serving with the Armed Forces feels unable to sign a certificate indicating fitness for a prospective event, it is proper for him to record that, at the time of his examination, the subject was or was not healthy.

Commercial enterprises and connections

8.25 A doctor should not associate himself with commerce in such a way as to let it influence, or appear to influence, his attitude towards the treatment of his patients. He must make it clear when writing a testimonial or commenting favourably on a commercial product to any manufacturer, especially one having any connection with medicine, that his name must not be used by the manufacturer for commercial purposes.

8.26 There should be no direct association of a doctor with any commercial enterprise engaged in the manufacture or sale of any substance which is claimed to be of value in the prevention or treatment of disease, and which is recommended to the public in such a fashion as to be calculated to encourage the practice of self-diagnosis and of self-medication or is of undisclosed nature or composition. Nor should a doctor be associated with any system or method of treatment which is not under medical control and which is advertised in the public press.

Undisclosed sharing of fees (dichotomy)

8.27 The secret division by two or more doctors of fees on a basis of commission, or some other defined method, is a practice that has brought the profession into disrepute on a number of occasions. Any undisclosed division of professional fees, save in a medical partnership publicly known to exist, is unethical.

Attendance upon colleagues

8.28 Every effort should be made to maintain the traditional practice of the medical profession whereby attendance by one doctor upon another or upon his dependants is without direct charge.

The doctor and his colleagues

Doctors in training

8.29 It is unethical to delegate any work to another doctor unless he is suitably qualified and experienced to undertake that work (for the General Medical Council's view, see 5.7 and 5.13). This principle applies to cross cover between specialties, to delegation to locums, and to delegation to junior staff within the same specialty. It applies to doctors working in general practice and, in so far as they are in personal working contact with people, to trainees in community medicine.

8.30 Provisional registration carries the same prescribing authority as full registration within the hospital where the doctor is employed. A fully registered practitioner is responsible for his actions to each patient. Principals in general practice and health authorities are responsible for the acts and omissions of those they employ.

8.31 A registered medical practitioner in training has a responsibility to his consultant or general practitioner trainer to take account of their advice to him. If he believes that the general advice he has been given is inapplicable to a particular situation or is not in the best interest of an individual patient he should seek further specific advice. If necessary he should ask the consultant or general practitioner to take back their delegated authority and take over the management of the patient's illness personally.

8.32 In other words, the primary responsibility of a junior doctor in a training post is to the patient and he should decline to do anything that he believes is not in the patient's best interests.

Deputising arrangements

8.33 Many requests for medical care are made outside normal working hours, but a doctor cannot be on duty continuously without detriment to the quality of his work and his health. Deputising arrangements must not jeopardise the welfare of the patient, so for deputising to be ethically acceptable two conditions must be satisfied. The doctor, who has been chosen and accepted by the patient, should ensure as far as practicable that the deputy is experienced, competent, conscientious and in other respects suitable to carry out the delegated responsibilities of the regular doctor. The patient's doctor must also ensure that communication and record systems are sufficient to permit proper treatment both during and after the deputising period.

8.34 In hospital practice it is the responsibility of the consultant to acquaint himself with the competence of his staff and to allow them to deputise only within their competence.

8.35 General practitioners who use a deputising service are effectively unable to exercise any direct choice of deputy and must rely on the management of the service to choose staff of appropriate competence. They have a duty, however, to inform the management of untoward incidents so that action can be taken to avoid any recurrence. Some deputising services are controlled solely by doctors, but most are controlled jointly by a commercial organisation and the profession. It has been customary in the past and obligatory since 1978, for there to be a professional advisory committee in connection with each deputising service to ensure maintenance of clinical and organisational standards and this should help principals using such services to feel satisfied that the deputies will be of an adequate standard.

Intra-professional disagreements

8.36 From time to time doctors working together in a practice or in the same locality find themselves in disagreement. It is important that disputes be resolved quickly and amicably within the profession itself. If animosities are allowed to fester they not only embitter local practice but also damage the reputation of the profession.

8.37 Most of these problems concern relationships based upon the traditions of the profession. Members of the BMA may obtain advice from their local division, or from the Association's Central Ethical Committee.

8.38 The ethical machinery of the BMA consists of the Central Ethical Committee itself, which is a standing committee of the Council, local ethical committees appointed by BMA divisions, and detailed uniform rules of procedure for the investigation of complaints. The preliminary stages for this machinery are that the complainant must write to the respondent (stating the complaint in terms sufficiently specific to enable the respondent to reply) intimating that he contemplates the initiation of a complaint through the ethical machinery of the Association, and inviting his reply. A copy of the letter of complaint, together with any reply, must be submitted to the Honorary Secretary of the appropriate Division of the Association. The Honorary Secretary then sends the correspondence to Head Office and obtains instructions on the steps to be taken to deal with the matter.

9 The doctor and the law

9.1 There is a close relationship between ethical and legal responsibilities. Though the ethical code does not, as in the civil law countries, form a branch of substantive law, there are a number of occasions when the ethical practice and the legal "standard of care" are inseparable (see also 6.3).

9.2 Before the passing of the *National Health Service Act 1946* medical law in England was dominated by the contractual relationship of doctor and patient. Apart from a number of specific statutory duties, such as the reporting of certain infectious diseases, doctors and surgeons tended to provide their services under direct contract to the patient. The jurisprudence which developed around the practice of medicine was largely derived from the law of contract. The Act of 1946 greatly modified this contractual relationship.

9.3 The National Health Service Acts consolidated in the Act of 1977 charge the Secretary of State with the overall responsibility to provide hospital, medical, and other allied services. The operation of the necessary supporting administrative structure and the changes brought by frequent parliamentary interventions, in addition to the flow of circulars from the Health Departments, account for the complexity of modern medical law.

9.4 This process has not in any way diminished the "legal standard" of patient care which is still best expressed as a duty to exercise reasonable care and skill. The position of the doctor in NHS practice, however, cannot be considered in isolation from his contractural obligations to the employing authority or Family Practitioner Committee, as the case may be.

9.5 The right to carry on medical practice is closely regulated under the Medical Acts 1858 to 1978. Until 1969 the General Medical Council had the power to erase from the *Register* the name of any fully or provisionally registered practitioner judged by the Disciplinary Committee of the Council to have been guilty of "infamous conduct in a professional respect". Undoubtedly this could have included a failure to conform to the ethical standards of the profession. *The Medical Act 1969* substituted the phrase "serious professional misconduct" for the expression quoted above.

Trends in medical legislation

9.6 Both at national and at European Community level, there continues to be legislative activity in various sectors of medicine.

9.7 In the United Kingdom children born as a result of artificial insemination by donor are illegitimate in the eyes of the law: the BMA has pressed for legislation to be prepared to enable children born as a result of AID, to which the husband or the mother has consented, to be defined as legitimate from the moment when conception is confirmed (see also 10.8).

Health of workers

9.8 Under statutory and regulatory legislation, the doctor engaged in occupational medicine is particularly likely to come into professional contact with workers. The Council of Ministers of the EEC wants to harmonise and improve the protective measures applying to workers in certain industries. One council directive, for example, attempts to improve the medical surveillance of workers in the vinyl chloride monomer and vinyl chloride polymer industry. Among other things, the directive prescribes that employers shall keep a register of workers who may be exposed to vinyl chloride monomer, with particulars of the type and duration of work and the exposure to which they have been subjected. The register is to be held by a doctor and a worker will be able, on request, to note the details about himself in the register.

9.9 A later article in the directive says that employers shall be required to ensure that the relevant workers are examined by a doctor both on recruitment or before taking up their activities, and subsequently. It is left to the member states of the EEC to determine how the registers and medical records are to be used for study and research purposes. (See also 1.20 for a discussion of medical records systems.)

10 Ethical dilemmas

10.1 Subjects discussed in this chapter fall into two broad categories. First, those dilemmas which continue to face the profession, but which have been the subject of considerable debate, and where a broad consensus of medical opinion favours a particular means of resolution in the majority of cases. Second, those dilemmas which are still the subject of widespread discussion about which no consensus view has been reached.

Consensus views

Termination of pregnancy (abortion)

10.2 The general principles enunciated in the *Statement on Therapeutic Abortion* by the World Medical Association in 1970, known as the Declaration of Oslo (reproduced in the Chapter on Ethical Codes and Statements) are broadly applicable to practice in the United Kingdom. However, legislation in different countries varies and the *Abortion Act 1967* has created problems for the doctor.

10.3 Because risk of injury to the health of a woman is statistically smaller if a pregnancy is terminated in the early months than if it is allowed to go to term, some people argue that abortion is justified if the woman requests it. But she needs a doctor to carry it out and the Act contains a "conscientious objection" clause by which the doctor can refuse to participate in treatment, though he has a duty to assist the patient to obtain alternative medical advice (and in the case of general practitioners in contract with a family practitioner committee the duty to indicate to the patient alternative sources of advice as part of the contract) if she wants it. There are three other problems arising from the 1967 Act and these are outlined in paragraphs 10.4 to 10.6.

10.4 The patient's immediate wishes may conflict with the doctor's judgment of her best long-term interests. If so, the doctor should be prepared to make arrangements for the patient to obtain a second opinion.

10.5 If a girl under the age of 16 requests termination without her parents' knowledge, the doctor may feel conflict between his duty to confidentiality and his responsibilities to the girl's parents or guardian. This cannot be resolved by any rigid code of practice. The

59

doctor should attempt to persuade the girl to allow him to inform her parents or guardian, but what he decides to do will depend upon his judgment of what is in the best interests of the patient.

10.6 The *Abortion Act 1967* specifically states that "nothing in the Act shall affect the provisions of the *Infant Life (Preservation) Act 1929*". This Act makes reference to a child "capable of being born alive". It further states that if a woman has been pregnant for 28 weeks or more it shall be *prima facie* proof that her child was capable of being born alive. However, it does *not* state that a child born before 28 weeks is not capable of being born alive and in fact such premature babies have sometimes survived. The doctor should recommend or perform termination after 20 weeks only if he is convinced that the health of the woman is seriously threatened, or if there is good reason to believe that the child will be seriously handicapped. If the doctor is uncertain he should always consult other colleagues, follow his own conscience, and act in the best interests of his patient.

10.7 Attempts have been made to amend the 1967 legislation, but at the present time 28 weeks remains the official period for legal viability of the foetus.

Artificial insemination by donor semen

10.8 Artificial insemination using semen from a donor raises a number of ethical problems. The doctor has a professional duty to consider the circumstances, in so far as they can be foreseen, of the child born as a result of successful inseminations. He cannot act merely as a technician; he should be satisfied that the people concerned have considered all the implications (see also 9.7).

Genetic counselling and investigation

10.9 The right to privacy in genetic counselling and research may be questioned because the individual affected may not be the only one who can benefit from medical advice. Certainty about an individual's genotype might affect his attitudes to life, and society's attitudes to him, with the possibility of considerable medical, economic and social repercussions. The problem occurs when one member of a family who is found to be carrying an abnormal gene is reluctant to allow this knowledge to be disseminated to other family members. Does the information belong solely to the individual in whom the abnormality was found, or does it, because of the shared nature of genetic material, belong to all the members of the family who could be affected?

10.10 The importance of such information probably outweighs the importance of complete individual medical confidentiality, providing that the information is kept to the medical profession and to those entitled to it because of their potential carrier state. Consideration must be given to informing the spouse, or potential spouse of a carrier, because he or she may bear some responsibility for passing such genes on to future generations.

Tissue transplantation

10.11 The profession is satisfied that the interests of live adult donors are adequately safeguarded by codes covering investigative and surgical procedures. Written consent should be obtained from the donor after a full explanation of the procedure involved and the possible consequences to him. The donor may also be advised to discuss the procedure with relatives, religious advisers, or anyone close to the patient, and these advisers should be able to meet the doctors if they wish.

10.12 There are probably no circumstances in which a child can be considered a suitable donor of non-regenerative tissue. There is no legal certainty about a parent's right to give consent on behalf of the child, but if this exists that right cannot extend to any procedure which is not in the child's best interests.

10.13 Bone marrow transplantation is an example of the donation of regenerative material. In many cases tissue comparability and the natural history of the disease means that the only suitable donor will be a child. In cases where a doctor considers the discomfort to a donor is minimal, it is not unethical to perform a bone marrow transplant with the consent of the parent. The procedure can be handled ethically only in the context of a compassionate and objective assessment of the individuals and families concerned, and the doctor must weigh up carefully the risk for the donor in reaching his final decision.

10.14 For the transplant of unpaired organs, the only possible donor is a dead person. Death may be certified after brain death, and the decision that brain death has occurred should be made by two or more doctors unconnected with the transplantation. One of these doctors should have been qualified for five years or more. The criteria laid down in paragraphs 28–30 of the Code of Practice "Cadaveric Organs for Transplantation" should be followed.

Jehovah's Witnesses and blood transfusion

10.15 When a Jehovah's Witness is suffering from a condition, the normal treatment for which may involve blood transfusion, the doctor should advise the patient of the usual treatment. If, as is probable, the patient refuses to consent to transfusion, the doctor must decide whether this caveat greatly increases the risk of the procedure. He must then reassess whether the risk from the disease outweighs the risk of the treatment without the ability to transfuse blood. The doctor may decide not to continue either because he believes that the possible benefits are outweighed by the potential dangers of the treatment, or because he is unwilling to have his options for management curtailed. If he declines further treatment for the latter reason he must refer the patient to a colleague who would be willing to undertake the case.

10.16 If the doctor decides to proceed with the treatment, he must honour his undertaking to the patient, having fully explained his concern about the results of withholding any part of the treatment.

10.17 When the child of a Jehovah's Witness requires a transfusion, the doctor can have the child made a ward of court or, if time does not allow, the doctor may proceed with the transfusion, having obtained the written agreement of a colleague supporting his opinion that the transfusion is necessary. The situation of the unborn child requiring an *in utero* transfusion remains unresolved.

No consensus: discussion continuing

Screening

10.18 Presymptomatic screening involves a departure from the traditional doctor-patient relationship and therefore has ethical implications. Has the medical profession any responsibility for "discovering" illness as distinct from responding to it when it presents itself? People believing themselves to be ill and presenting for treatment are only a proportion of the ill people within the community. Some are unwell but do not seek medical help; others do not know that they are ill. The ethical dilemma lies in the fact that screening could reveal many sick persons who do not at present seek medical help.

10.19 Before embarking on a screening programme (other than as a research procedure) a doctor must satisfy himself that:

   (*a*) the individuals in a given population wish to know whether they have the disease for which the screening is proposed.

(b) the screening techniques he will use are reliable and will not give an unacceptable level of false negatives or false positives.

(c) medical science has the ability, and the population the financial resources, to provide such practical assistance as is currently available.

10.20 In considering the financial implications the doctor should remember that it will be some time before the cost of the screening programme is offset by the benefits accrued from earlier diagnosis of the disease.

Severely malformed infants

10.21 A malformed infant has the same rights as a normal infant. It follows that ordinary non-medical care which is necessary for the maintenance of the life of a normal infant should not be withheld from a malformed infant.

10.22 Where medical or surgical measures might be needed to preserve the life of a severely malformed infant, every opportunity should be taken for deliberation and discussion, as time permits. This requires the closest co-operation between the doctor in charge, the parents of the child, and any colleagues whose opinion is felt to be helpful, including the patient's general practitioner. The doctors have a particular duty to ensure that parents have as full an understanding as possible of the options and the likely outcome, with or without surgery or other means of active intervention.

10.23 The parents of an infant born severely malformed must never be left with the feeling that they are having to exercise their responsibility to make decisions regarding consent to the management of their child without help and understanding. They should be encouraged to seek advice from anyone in whose judgment they have faith. The doctor in charge is responsible for the initiation or the withholding of treatment in the best interests of the infant. He must attend primarily to the needs and rights of the individual infant, and he must also have concern for the family as a whole.

10.24 If doubts persist in the minds either of the parents or doctor in charge as to the best interests of the infant, a second medical opinion should be sought.

10.25 In emergencies there may be no time for consultation with parents or anyone else, and the doctor in charge must exercise his clinical judgment.

Terminal illness and death

10.26 The word "euthanasia", literally meaning "gentle and easy death", has not been used as the title for this section since the complications resulting from new techniques of life support systems have opened up new areas of ethical dilemmas which are not strictly covered by this term.

10.27 The duty of a doctor to ensure that a patient dies with dignity and as little suffering as possible remains unchanged. The possibility of maintaining "physiological life", that is, the continuation of the body functions by artificial means, whilst the patient remains unconscious over a period of months and possibly years, has introduced a new dimension into the debate—"quality of life". Clearly the sustaining of physiological functions with no prospect of recovery of consciousness or contact with the patient's environment has led to considerable debate as to whether or not such support systems should be continued, and who should be reponsible for the decision to turn off such systems. Views vary widely from those who consider that all support must continue to others who feel that such support systems should not be used in certain circumstances. Several States in the USA have legislation permitting a patient to express his wishes in a "will to life" declaration when he is in good bodily and mental health. This debate will clearly continue for some time. The doctor's basic duty is to preserve life and there is no rigid code by which such considerations as "quality of life" can be considered when deciding appropriate treatment.

10.28 The word "euthanasia" has been further complicated by its interpretation as "mercy killing".

10.29 The literal meaning of euthanasia—"gentle and easy death"—carries no ethical difficulties for a doctor. Indeed, the doctor has a responsibility to ensure that his patient dies with dignity and as little suffering as possible. The second meaning— "mercy killing"—calls for further comment. The position is now complicated by the application of "compulsory", "voluntary", "active" and "passive" to euthanasia. In no country is euthanasia legal. Voluntary euthanasia bills were defeated in Parliament in 1936, 1969 and 1976.

10.30 *Compulsory* euthanasia—meaning a decision by society that an individual, either against his will or without being able to consent, should have his life terminated—is totally abhorrent to the medical profession.

10.31 *Voluntary* euthanasia—in which an individual, either in advance or at the time but in full control of his faculties, expresses a wish that in certain circumstances his life should be terminated—does have followers and there are associations for its promotion.

10.32 The distinction between *active* euthanasia, in which drugs are given, or other procedures carried out to cause death, and *passive* euthanasia, in which drugs or other procedures which might prolong life are withheld, generally applies to voluntary euthanasia. Some people regard passive euthanasia as simply not interfering with the course of nature. The argument may be complicated by the ethics of giving drugs, such as analgesics, in increasing doses and thus indirectly shortening life.

10.33 Doctors vary in their approach to passive euthanasia but the profession condemns legalised active voluntary euthanasia.

Brain death

10.34 In October 1976 the Conference of Medical Royal Colleges and their Faculties in the United Kingdom published a report expressing the opinion that "brain death" could be diagnosed with certainty. A subsequent report by the Conference of 15 January 1979 concluded that the identification of brain death means that the patient is dead, whether or not the function of some organs, such as a heart beat, is still maintained by artificial means (see Chapter on Ethical Codes and Statements). Termination of the artificial support, therefore, is not an act of euthanasia.

Reduction of services to patients

10.35 The obligation not to damage care for actual patients and to refuse to work under inadequate conditions is strengthened by the doctor's necessary authority as the person identifiably responsible for the management of the patient's illness.

10.36 The doctor must decide whether or not conditions are adequate for him to provide care of patients. Refusal by a doctor to work for patients on the grounds that adequate conditions are lacking is not industrial action but the performance of his duties. He does not stop his work by refusing to proceed with the care of patients, since it is part of his practice continuously to exercise his judgment as to the adequacy of conditions for diagnostic and therapeutic work. Such refusals to proceed, so far from being action *against* patients, as they are sometimes perceived as being, constitute in fact, action *on behalf of* the patient (see also 5.2).

10.37 Where the State is responsible for providing the bulk of health care in a social security system, it is difficult to reach any conclusion other than that the State and the profession in these circumstances have a peculiar obligation to one another. The profession should not require the State to renegue on its social responsibilities and the State should not require doctors to renegue on their ethical responsibilities. (See the Charter of Nuremburg reproduced in the Chapter on Ethical Codes and Statements.)

10.38 The dilemma that exists and seems likely to persist is that the two sets of responsibilities are occasionally incompatible, if not in direct conflict. For example, the profession may justifiably think that it has an ethical responsibility to provide the best available treatment, while the State may regard itself as being responsible to the community to limit the resources available to the National Health Service on criteria other than the needs of patients. With this type of conflict one or other view cannot be sustained, and each individual is thrown back on his own ethic to determine what action he will take.

10.39 Doctors hold widely differing views about withdrawal of their services. Certain material resources necessary for the treatment of patients may not be available to the doctor, and opinions will differ as to when the circumstances justify such action, if at all.

10.40 Withdrawal of services from a monopoly employer has much greater consequences for the community than withdrawal of services from a near-monopoly employer or from one of a number of competing employers, since in the former case no alternative exists to provide even an emergency supply. Within a monopoly NHS doctors could not treat patients outside it, and would therefore find themselves totally prevented by their ethical responsibilities from even a temporary withdrawal of services. Such a situation would present the ethical dilemma at its most critical.

10.41 The overall professional ethic of bringing relief to the sick remains unchanged and the Representative Body of the BMA clearly had this in mind when it passed the following resolution in 1979: "That this Meeting unequivocally condemns the kind of industrial action which increases the sum of human suffering".

10.42 It will remain the duty of the doctor to decide, according to his own conscience, what action he will take. He must bear in mind the basic ethical duties of a doctor and the view of the profession in the UK as expressed in the above resolution.

Allocation of resources within the NHS

10.43 Within the National Health Service resources are finite, and this may restrict the freedom of the doctor to advise his patient, who will usually be unaware of the limitation. This situation infringes the ordinary relationship between patient and doctor, described in Chapter 2. Some of the situations which may arise are discussed briefly.

10.44 The resources made available to the NHS by Parliament can never be infinite. Patients will seek advice in situations where the doctor believes treatment to be desirable; however, because of limitation of resources, such treatment may not be available at that time or place within the NHS. The doctor has a duty to explain the position to the patient, including an assessment of any medical implications of delay, unless it is not in the patient's interests to be made aware of the risks of delay. Should the patient request a second opinion, or an opinion in different circumstances, the doctor should assist him in obtaining such an opinion.

10.45 If, as a result of resources restriction, the overall conditions in which a doctor is required to practise within the NHS fall below a minimal level of acceptability to the doctor, he may feel that it would be unethical to continue to advise patients in a situation where his ability to offer treatment is curtailed through no fault of his own. As the resources available within the NHS are limited, the doctor has a general duty to advise on their equitable allocation and efficient utilisation. This duty is subordinate to his professional duty to the individual who seeks his clinical advice. It is clearly the ethical duty of the doctor to use the most economic and efficacious treatment available.

11 Ethical codes and statements

The Hippocratic Oath

The methods and details of medical practice change with the passage of time and the advance of knowledge. However, many fundamental principles of professional behaviour have remained unaltered through the recorded history of medicine. The Hippocratic Oath was probably written in the 5th century BC, and was intended to be affirmed by each doctor on entry to the medical profession. In translation it reads as follows:

> I swear by Apollo the physician, and Aesculapius and Health, and All-heal, and all the gods and goddesses, that, according to my ability and judgment, I will keep this Oath and this stipulation—to reckon him who taught me this Art equally dear to me as my parents, to share my substance with him, and relieve his necessities if required; to look upon his offspring in the same footing as my own brothers, and to teach them this Art, if they shall wish to learn it, without fee or stipulation; and that by precept, lecture and every other mode of instruction, I will impart a knowledge of the Art to my own sons, and those of my teachers, and to disciples bound by a stipulation and oath according to the law of medicine, but to none other. I will follow that system of regimen which, according to my ability and judgment, I consider for the benefit of my patients, and abstain from whatever is deleterious and mischievous. I will give no deadly medicine to anyone if asked, nor suggest any such counsel; and in like manner I will not give to a woman a pessary to produce abortion. With purity and with holiness I will pass my life and practise my Art. I will not cut persons labouring under the stone, but will leave this to be done by men who are practitioners of this work. Into whatever houses I enter, I will go into them for the benefit of the sick, and will abstain from every voluntary act of mischief and corruption; and, further, from the seduction of females, or males, of freemen or slaves. Whatever, in connection with my professional practice, or not in connection with it, I see or hear, in the life of men, which ought not to be spoken of abroad, I will not divulge, as reckoning that all such should be kept secret. While I continue to keep this Oath unviolated, may it be granted to me to

enjoy life and the practice of the Art, respected by all men, in all times. But should I trespass and violate this Oath, may the reverse be my lot.

The World Medical Association

International Code of Medical Ethics

One of the first acts of the World Medical Association, when formed in 1947, was to produce a modern restatement of the Hippocratic Oath, known as the Declaration of Geneva, and to base upon it an International Code of Medical Ethics which applies both in times of peace and war. The Declaration of Geneva, as amended by the 22nd World Medical Assembly, Sydney, Australia, in August 1968 and the 35th World Medical Assembly, Venice, Italy, in October 1983, reads:

At the time of being admitted as a Member of the Medical Profession:

I solemnly pledge myself to consecrate my life to the service of humanity;
I will give to my teachers the respect and gratitude which is their due;
I will practise my profession with conscience and dignity;
The health of my patient will be my first consideration;
I will respect the secrets which are confided in me, even after the patient has died;
I will maintain by all the means in my power, the honour and the noble traditions of the medical profession;
My colleagues will be my brothers;
I will not permit considerations of religion, nationality, race, party politics or social standing to intervene between my duty and my patients;
I will maintain the utmost respect for human life from its beginning even under threat and I will not use my medical knowledge contrary to the laws of humanity;
I make these promises solemnly, freely and upon my honour.

The English text of the International Code of Medical Ethics is as follows:

Duties of physicians in general
A PHYSICIAN SHALL always maintain the highest standards of

professional conduct.

A PHYSICIAN SHALL not permit motives of profit to influence the free and independent exercise of professional judgment on behalf of patients.

A PHYSICIAN SHALL, in all types of medical practice, be dedicated to providing competent medical service in full technical and moral independence, with compassion and respect for human dignity.

A PHYSICIAN SHALL deal honestly with patients and colleagues, and strive to expose those physicians deficient in character or competence, or who engage in fraud or deception.

The following practices are deemed to be unethical conduct:

(a) Self advertising by physicians, unless permitted by the laws of the country and the Code of Ethics of the National Medical Association.

(b) Paying or receiving any fee or any other consideration solely to procure the referral of a patient or for prescribing or referring a patient to any source.

A PHYSICIAN SHALL respect the rights of patients, of colleagues, and of other health professionals, and shall safeguard patient confidences.

A PHYSICIAN SHALL act only in the patient's interest when providing medical care which might have the effect of weakening the physical and mental condition of the patient.

A PHYSICIAN SHALL use great caution in divulging discoveries or new techniques or treatment through non-professional channels.

A PHYSICIAN SHALL certify only that which he has personally verified.

Duties of physicians to the sick

A PHYSICIAN SHALL always bear in mind the obligation of preserving human life.

A PHYSICIAN SHALL owe his patients complete loyalty and all the resources of his science. Whenever an examination or treatment is beyond the physician's capacity he should summon another physician who has the necessary ability.

A PHYSICIAN SHALL preserve absolute confidentiality on all he knows about his patient even after the patient has died.

A PHYSICIAN SHALL give emergency care as a humanitarian duty unless he is assured that others are willing and able to give such care.

Duties of physicians to each other

A PHYSICIAN SHALL behave towards his colleagues as he would

have them behave towards him.

A PHYSICIAN SHALL NOT entice patients from his colleagues.

A PHYSICIAN SHALL observe the principles of "The Declaration of Geneva" approved by the World Medical Association.

Subsequently, the World Medical Association has considered and published material on a number of ethical matters.

Discrimination in medicine

The following motion on the subject of discrimination in medicine was adopted by the World Medical Association in 1973:

> "WHEREAS: The Declaration of Geneva, adopted and published by the World Medical Association, states, *inter alia,* that, 'I (a medical practitioner) WILL NOT PERMIT considerations of religion, nationality, race, party politics or social standing to intervene between my duty and my patient';
>
> THEREFORE, BE IT RESOLVED by the 27th World Medical Assembly meeting in Munich, that the World Medical Association *vehemently condemns* colour, political and religious discrimination of any form in the training of medical practitioners and in the practice of medicine and in the provision of health services for the peoples of the world."

Rights of the patient

In 1981 the World Medical Association adopted a Statement on the rights of the patient. Known as the Declaration of Lisbon, it reads:

> Recognizing that there may be practical, ethical or legal difficulties, a physician should always act according to his/her conscience and always in the best interest of the patient. The following Declaration represents some of the principal rights which the medical profession seeks to provide to patients.
>
> Whenever legislation or government action denies these rights of the patient, physicians should seek by appropriate means to assure or to restore them.
>
> (*a*) The patient has the right to choose his physician freely.
>
> (*b*) The patient has the right to be cared for by a physician who is free to make clinical and ethical judgements without any outside interference.
>
> (*c*) The patient has the right to accept or to refuse treatment after

receiving adequate information.

(d) The patient has the right to expect that his physician will respect the confidential nature of all his medical and personal details.

(e) The patient has the right to die in dignity.

(f) The patient has the right to receive or to decline spiritual and moral comfort including the help of a minister of an appropriate religion.

Human experimentation

In 1964, the World Medical Association drew up a code of ethics on human experimentation. This code, known as the Declaration of Helsinki, as amended by the 29th World Medical Assembly, Helsinki, Finland, in 1975, and by the 35th World Medical Assembly, Venice, Italy, in 1983, reads:

> It is the mission of the medical doctor to safeguard the health of the people. His or her knowledge and conscience are dedicated to the fulfilment of this mission.
>
> The Declaration of Geneva of the World Medical Association binds the physician with the words, "The health of my patient will be my first consideration", and the International Code of Medical Ethics declares that "A physician shall act only in the patient's interest when providing medical care which might have the effect of weakening the physical and mental condition of the patient."
>
> The purpose of biomedical research involving human subjects must be to improve diagnostic, therapeutic and prophylactic procedures and the understanding of the aetiology and pathogenesis of disease.
>
> In current medical practice most diagnostic, therapeutic or prophylactic procedures involve hazards. This applies especially to biomedical research.
>
> Medical progress is based on research which ultimately must rest in part on experimentation involving human subjects.
>
> In the field of biomedical research a fundamental distinction must be recognised between medical research in which the aim is essentially diagnostic or therapeutic for a patient, and medical research, the essential object of which is purely scientific and without implying direct diagnostic or therapeutic value to the person subjected to the research.
>
> Special caution must be exercised in the conduct of research

which may affect the environment, and the welfare of animals used for research must be respected.

Because it is essential that the results of laboratory experiments be applied to human beings to further scientific knowledge and to help suffering humanity, the World Medical Association has prepared the following recommendations as a guide to every physician in biomedical research involving human subjects. They should be kept under review in the future. It must be stressed that the standards as drafted are only a guide to physicians all over the world. Physicians are not relieved from criminal, civil and ethical responsibilities under the laws of their own countries.

I *Basic principles*

(1) Biomedical research involving human subjects must conform to generally accepted scientific principles and should be based on adequately performed laboratory and animal experimentation and on a thorough knowledge of the scientific literature.

(2) The design and performance of each experimental procedure involving human subjects should be clearly formulated in an experimental protocol which should be transmitted to a specially appointed independent committee for consideration, comment and guidance.

(3) Biomedical research involving human subjects should be conducted only by scientifically qualified persons and under the supervision of a clinically competent medical person. The responsibility for the human subject must always rest with the medically qualified person and never rest on the subject of the research, even though the subject has given his or her consent.

(4) Biomedical research involving human subjects cannot legitimately be carried out unless the importance of the objective is in proportion to the inherent risk to the subject.

(5) Every biomedical research project involving human subjects should be preceded by careful assessment of predictable risks in comparison with foreseeable benefits to the subject or to others. Concern for the interests of the subject must always prevail over the interests of science and society.

(6) The right of the research subject to safeguard his or her integrity must always be respected. Every precaution should be taken to respect the privacy of the subject and to minimize the impact of the study on the subject's physical and mental integrity and on the personality of the subject.

(7) Physicians should abstain from engaging in research projects

74

involving human subjects unless they are satisfied that the hazards involved are believed to be predictable. Physicians should cease any investigation if the hazards are found to outweigh the potential benefits.

(8) In publication of the results of his or her research, the physician is obliged to preserve the accuracy of the results. Reports of experimentation not in accordance with the principles laid down in this Declaration should not be accepted for publication.

(9) In any research on human beings, each potential subject must be adequately informed of the aims, methods, anticipated benefits and potential hazards of the study and the discomfort it may entail. He or she should be informed that he or she is at liberty to abstain from participation in the study and that he or she is free to withdraw his or her consent to participation at any time. The physician should then obtain the subject's freely-given informed consent, preferably in writing.

(10) When obtaining informed consent for the research project the physician should be particularly cautious if the subject is in a dependent relationship to him or her or may consent under duress. In that case the informed consent should be obtained by a physician who is not engaged in the investigation and who is completely independent of this official relationship.

(11) In case of legal incompetence, informed consent should be obtained from the legal guardian in accordance with national legislation. Where physical or mental incapacity makes it impossible to obtain informed consent, or when the subject is a minor, permission from the responsible relative replaces that of the subject in accordance with national legislation.

Whenever the minor child is in fact able to give a consent, the minor's consent must be obtained in addition to the consent of the minor's legal guardian.

(12) The research protocol should always contain a statement of the ethical considerations involved and should indicate that the principles enunciated in the present Declaration are complied with.

II *Medical research combined with professional care*
(Clinical research)

(1) In the treatment of the sick person, the physician must be free to use a new diagnostic and therapeutic measure, if in his or her judgment it offers hope of saving life, re-establishing health or

alleviating suffering.

(2) The potential benefits, hazards and discomfort of a new method should be weighed against the advantages of the best current diagnostic and therapeutic methods.

(3) In any medical study, every patient—including those of a control group, if any—should be assured of the best proven diagnostic and therapeutic method.

(4) The refusal of the patient to participate in a study must never interfere with the physician-patient relationship.

(5) If the physician considers it essential not to obtain informed consent, the specific reasons for this proposal should be stated in the experimental protocol for transmission to the independent committee (I.2).

(6) The physician can combine medical research with professional care, the objective being the acquisition of new medical knowledge, only to the extent that medical research is justified by its potential diagnostic or therapeutic value for the patient.

III *Non-therapeutic biomedical research involving human subjects (Non-clinical biomedical research)*

(1) In the purely scientific application of medical research carried out on a human being, it is the duty of the physician to remain the protector of the life and health of that person on whom biomedical research is being carried out.

(2) The subjects should be volunteers—either healthy persons or patients for whom the experimental design is not related to the patient's illness.

(3) The investigator or the investigating team should discontinue the research if in his/her or their judgment it may, if continued, be harmful to the individual.

(4) In research on man, the interest of science and society should never take precedence over considerations related to the well-being of the subject.

Therapeutic abortion

In 1970 the World Medical Association drew up a Statement on Therapeutic Abortion. This code, known as the Declaration of Oslo, was amended by the 35th World Medical Assembly, Venice, Italy, in October 1983, and states:

(1) The first moral principle imposed upon the physician is

76

respect for human life from its beginning.

(2) Circumstances which bring the vital interests of a mother into conflict with the vital interests of her unborn child create a dilemma and raise the question whether or not the pregnancy should be deliberately terminated.

(3) Diversity of response to this situation results from the diversity of attitudes towards the life of the unborn child. This is a matter of individual conviction and conscience which must be respected.

(4) It is not the role of the medical profession to determine the attitudes and rules of any particular state or community in this matter, but it is our duty to attempt both to ensure the protection of our patients and to safeguard the rights of the physician within society.

(5) Therefore, where the law allows therapeutic abortion to be performed, the procedure should be performed by a physician competent to do so in premises approved by the appropriate authority.

(6) If the physician considers that his convictions do not allow him to advise or perform an abortion, he may withdraw while ensuring the continuity of (medical) care by a qualified colleague.

(7) This statement, while it is endorsed by the General Assembly of the World Medical Association, is not to be regarded as binding on any individual member association unless it is adopted by that member association.

Medical secrecy

The following Resolution on "Medical secrecy" was adopted by the World Medical Association in 1973:

"WHEREAS: The privacy of the individual is highly prized in most societies and widely accepted as a civil right; and

WHEREAS: The confidential nature of the patient-doctor relationship is regarded by most doctors as extremely important and is taken for granted by the patient; and

WHEREAS: There is an increasing tendency towards an intrusion on medical secrecy;

THEREFORE BE IT RESOLVED that the 27th World Medical Assembly reaffirm the vital importance of maintaining medical secrecy not as a privilege for the doctor, but to protect the privacy of the individual as the basis for the confidential relationship between the patient and his doctor; and ask the United Nations, representing the people of the world, to give to the medical profession the needed help and to show ways for securing this fundamental right for the individual human being."

Use of computers in medicine

The following statement, adopted by the World Medical Assembly in 1973, was amended by the 35th World Medical Assembly in Venice, Italy, in October 1983, and reads:

The World Medical Association, having taken note of the great advances and advantages resulting from the use of computers and electronic data processing in the field of health, especially in patient care and epidemiology, makes the following recommendations:

(1) National medical associations should take all possible steps to ensure the privacy, the security and confidentiality of information on their patients;

(2) It is not a breach of confidentiality to release or transfer confidential health care information required for the purpose of conducting scientific research, management audits, financial audits, program evaluations, or similar studies, provided the information released does not identify, directly or indirectly, any individual patient in any report of such research, audit or evaluation, or otherwise disclose patient identities in any manner;

(3) National medical associations should oppose any effort to enact legislation on electronic data processing which could endanger or undermine the right of the patient to privacy, security and confidentiality. Effective safeguards against unauthorized use or retransmission of social security numbers and other personal information must be assured before such information enters the computer;

(4) Medical data banks should never be linked to other central data banks.

Torture and other cruel, inhuman or degrading treatment or punishment

In 1975 the World Medical Association adopted the following guidelines for medical doctors concerning Torture and Other Cruel, Inhuman or Degrading Treatment or Punishment in relation to Detention and Imprisonment (Declaration of Tokyo):

78

It is the privilege of the medical doctor to practise medicine in the service of humanity, to preserve and restore bodily and mental health without distinction as to persons, to comfort and to ease the suffering of his or her patients. The utmost respect for human life is to be maintained even under threat, and no use made of any medical knowledge contrary to the laws of humanity.

For the purpose of this Declaration, torture is defined as the deliberate, systematic or wanton infliction of physical or mental suffering by one or more persons acting alone or on the orders of any authority, to force another person to yield information, to make a confession, or for any other reason.

Declaration

(1) The doctor shall not countenance, condone or participate in the practice of torture or other forms of cruel, inhuman or degrading procedures, whatever the offence of which the victim of such procedures is suspected, accused or guilty, and whatever the victim's beliefs or motives, and in all situations, including armed conflict and civil strife.

(2) The doctor shall not provide any premises, instruments, substances or knowledge to facilitate the practice of torture or other forms of cruel, inhuman or degrading treatment or to diminish the ability of the victim to resist such treatment.

(3) The doctor shall not be present during any procedure during which torture or other forms of cruel, inhuman or degrading treatment is used or threatened.

(4) A doctor must have complete clinical independence in deciding upon the care of a person for whom he or she is medically responsible. The doctor's fundamental role is to alleviate the distress of his or her fellow men, and no motive, whether personal, collective or political, shall prevail against this higher purpose.

(5) Where a prisoner refuses nourishment and is considered by the doctor as capable of forming an unimpaired and rational judgment concerning the consequences of such a voluntary refusal of nourishment, he or she shall not be fed artificially. The decision as to the capacity of the prisoner to form such a judgment should be confirmed by at least one other independent doctor. The consequences of the refusal of nourishment shall be explained by the doctor to the prisoner.

(6) The World Medical Association will support, and should encourage the international community, the national medical

associations and fellow doctors, to support the doctor and his or her family in the face of threats or reprisals resulting from a refusal to condone the use of torture or other forms of cruel, inhuman or degrading treatment.

Terminal Illness

In 1983 the World Medical Association adopted a statement on Terminal Illness (Declaration of Venice), which reads:

(1) The duty of the physician is to heal and, where possible, relieve suffering and act to protect the best interests of his patients.

(2) There shall be no exception to this principle even in the case of incurable disease or malformation.

(3) This principle does not preclude application of the following rules:

3.1 The physician may relieve suffering of a terminally ill patient by withholding treatment with the consent of the patient or his immediate family if unable to express his will.

Withholding of treatment does not free the physician from his obligation to assist the dying person and give him the necessary medicaments to mitigate the terminal phase of his illness.

3.2 The physician shall refrain from employing any extraordinary means which would prove of no benefit for the patient.

3.3 The physician may, when the patient cannot reverse the final process of cessation of vital functions, apply such artificial means as are necessary to keep organs active for trans-plantation provided he acts in accordance with the laws of the country or by virtue of a formal consent given by the responsible person and provided the certification of death or the irreversibility of vital activity had been made by physicians unconnected with the transplantation and the patient receiving treatment. These artificial means shall not be paid for by the donor or his relatives. Physicians treating the donor shall be totally independent of those treating the recipient and of the recipient himself.

Statements on death

World Medical Association

The World Medical Association formulated a Statement on Death in 1968. Known as the Declaration of Sydney, it was amended by the 35th World Medical Assembly in Venice, Italy, in 1983, and reads:

(1) The determination of the time of death is in most countries the legal responsibility of the physician and should remain so. Usually the physician will be able without special assistance to decide that a person is dead, employing the classical criteria known to all physicians.

(2) Two modern practices in medicine, however, have made it necessary to study the question of the time of death further: (a) the ability to maintain by artificial means the circulation of oxygenated blood through tissues of the body which may have been irreversibly injured and (b) the use of cadaver organs such as heart or kidneys for transplantation.

(3) A complication is that death is a gradual process at the cellular level with tissues varying in their ability to withstand deprivation of oxygen. But clinical interest lies not in the state of preservation of isolated cells but in the fate of a person. Here the point of death of the different cells and organs is not so important as the certainty that the process has become irreversible by whatever techniques of resuscitation that may be employed.

(4) It is essential to determine the irreversible cessation of all functions of the entire brain, including the brain stem. This determination will be based on clinical judgment supplemented if necessary by a number of diagnostic aids. However, no single technological criterion is entirely satisfactory in the present state of medicine nor can any one technological procedure be substituted for the overall judgment of the physician. If transplantation of an organ is involved, the decision that death exists should be made by two or more physicians and the physicians determining the moment of death should in no way be immediately concerned with the performance of the transplantation.

(5) Determination of the point of death of the person makes it ethically permissible to cease attempts at resuscitation and in countries where the law permits, to remove organs from the cadaver provided that prevailing legal requirements of consent have been fulfilled.

Conference of Medical Royal Colleges

The following Memorandum was issued by the Honorary Secretary of the Conference of Medical Royal Colleges and their Faculties in the United Kingdom on 15 January 1979:

(1) In October 1976 the Conference of Royal Colleges and their Faculties (UK) published a report unanimously expressing the opinion that "brain death", when it had occurred, could be diagnosed with certainty. The report has been widely accepted. The conference was not at that time asked whether or not it believed that death itself should be presumed to occur when brain death takes place or whether it would come to some other conclusion. The present report examines this point and should be considered as an addendum to the original report.

(2) Exceptionally, as a result of massive trauma, death occurs instantaneously or near-instantaneously. Far more commonly, death is not an event: it is a process, the various organs and systems supporting the continuation of life failing and eventually ceasing altogether to function, successively and at different times.

(3) Cessation of respiration and cessation of the heart beat are examples of organic failure occurring during the process of dying, and since the moment that the heart beat ceases is usually detectable with simplicity by no more than clinical means, it has for many centuries been accepted as the moment of death itself, without any serious attempt being made to assess the validity of this assumption.

(4) It is now universally accepted, by the lay public as well as by the medical profession, that it is not possible to equate death itself with the cessation of the heart beat. Quite apart from the elective cardiac arrest of open-heart surgery, spontaneous cardiac arrest followed by successful resuscitation is today a commonplace, and although the more sensational accounts of occurrences of this kind still refer to the patient being "dead" until restoration of the heart beat, the use of the quote marks usually demonstrates that this word is not to be taken literally, for to most people the one aspect of death that is beyond debate is its irreversibility.

(5) In the majority of cases in which a dying patient passes through the processes leading to the irreversible state we call death, successive organic failures eventually reach a point at which brain death occurs and this is the point of no return.

(6) In a minority of cases brain death does not occur as a result of the failure of other organs or systems but as a direct result of severe damage to the brain itself from, perhaps, a head injury or a spontaneous intracranial haemorrhage. Here the order of events is

82

reversed; instead of the failure of such vital functions as heart beat and respiration eventually resulting in brain death, brain death results in the cessation of spontaneous respiration; this is normally followed within minutes by cardiac arrest due to hypoxia. If, however, oxygenation is maintained by artificial ventilation the heart beat can continue for some days, and haemoperfusion will for a time be adequate to maintain function in other organs, such as the liver and kidneys.

(7) Whatever the mode of its production, brain death represents the stage at which a patient becomes truly dead, because by then all functions of the brain have permanently and irreversibly ceased. It is not difficult or illogical in any way to equate this with the concept in many religions of the departure of the spirit from the body.

(8) In the majority of cases, since brain death is part of or the culmination of a failure of all vital functions, there is no necessity for a doctor specifically to identify brain death individually before concluding that the patient is dead. In a minority of cases in which it is brain death that causes failure of other organs and systems, the fact that these systems can be artificially maintained even after brain death has made it important to establish a diagnostic routine which will identify with certainty the existence of brain death.

Conclusion

(9) It is the conclusion of the Conference that the identification of brain death means that the patient is dead, whether or not the function of some organs, such as heart beat, is still maintained by artificial means.

The Commonwealth Medical Association

The following Ethical Code of the Commonwealth Medical Association was approved at its meeting in Jamaica in 1974:

(1) The doctor's primary loyalty is to his patient.

(2) His vocation and skill shall be devoted to the amelioration of symptoms, the cure of illness, and the promotion of health.

(3) He shall respect human life and studiously avoid doing it injury.

(4) He shall share all the knowledge he may have gained with his colleagues without any reserve.

(5) He shall respect the confidence of his patient as he would his own.

(6) He shall by precept and example maintain the dignity and ideals of the profession, and permit no bias based on race, creed or socio-economic factors to affect his professional practice.

Note: The word "patient" used in this Code embraces the prisoner or other persons whom a doctor might be called upon to attend at another's bidding.

Standing Committee of Doctors of the EEC

The Standing Committee of Doctors of the EEC adopted the following Declaration concerning the practice of medicine within the Community at its plenary Assembly Session held in Nuremberg in November 1967 (Charter of Nuremburg (orig. French)). The text is as published in *The Handbook of Policy Statements 1959–1982*, Standing Committee of Doctors of the EEC.

(1) Every man must be free to choose his doctor.

Every man must be guaranteed that whatever a doctor's obligations vis-à-vis society, whatever he confides to his doctor and to those assisting him will remain secret.

Every man must have a guarantee that the doctor he consults is morally and technically totally independent and that he has free choice of therapy.

Human life from its beginning and the human person in its integrity, both material and spiritual, must be the object of total respect.

Guarantees of these rights for patients imply a health policy resulting from firm agreement between those responsible to the State and the organised medical profession.

(2) The aim common to the health policy of states and medical practice is to protect the health of all its citizens.

It is the duty of States to take all precautions to ensure all social classes—without discrimination—have access to all the medical care they require. Every man has the right to obtain from the social institutions and the medical corps the help he needs to preserve, develop or recover his health: he has an obligation to contribute materially and morally to these objectives.

Economic expansion finds one of its principal human justifications in the advancement of resources allocated to health; the medical profession intends to do all in its power to increase, at equal cost, the human and social effectiveness of medicine.

(3) The unusual necessary contact between the doctor and his patient takes account of the fact that these two partners belong to one community, a condition of all health and social policy. But there must be reciprocal confidence between the patient and his doctor based on the certitude that in his treatment the doctor holds in the highest esteem and has consciously consecrated all his knowledge to the service of the human person. No matter what his method of practice or remuneration the doctor must have access to the existing resources necessary for medical intervention; he must have free choice of decision bearing in mind the interests of his patient and the concrete possibilities offered by the advancements of science and medical techniques.

Doctors must be free to organise their practice together in a manner complying with the technical and social needs of the profession, on condition that moral and technical independence be respected and the personal responsibility of each practitioner maintained.

(4) Whatever its method of practice, the medical profession is one. These methods are complementary. They derive from the same deontology although they may be submitted to different organisational conditions. Respect for moral laws and for the basic principles of medical practice is assured by independent institutions, emanating from the Medical Corps and invested, particularly under the highest judicial processes in the country, with disciplinary and judicial power.

Every doctor has a moral obligation to actively participate in his professional organisation. Through this organisation he participates in the elaboration of the country's health policy.

Members of the profession can and must fight for respect of basic principles in the practice of medicine, on condition that the rights of the patient are safeguarded.

(5) Hospital equipment must be within the compass of its specific mission in the service of the whole population. Its establishment is the result of a planned policy in which the public powers and the organised profession participate, allocating to public power and private initiative fuller distribution of health establishments. It comprises a variety of establishments, graded and co-ordinated among themselves, meeting the task or several tasks given to it:

prevention, care, rehabilitation, teaching, research. . . . This organisation as a whole must take into consideration the principles given in the hospital charter drawn up by the Standing Committee of Doctors of the EEC and respect the autonomy of each establishment which must entail administrative and medical direction. The professional independence of the hospital doctor must be guaranteed by unquestionable criteria of nomination and a statute assuring him stability of function, economic independence and social protection.

"Technical progress, the basis of our industrial civilisation, and economic expansion which is its fruit, have for their natural end, especially thanks to a health policy, to bring about full physical and spiritual development of man, of all men."

European Union of General Practitioners (UEMO)

The European Union of General Practitioners (UEMO) adopted the following statement on Medical Confidentiality in Relation to the use of Modern Methods of Communication (EDP) in Medicine at Amsterdam in May 1979:

The patient has a right to expect that his doctor will maintain professional confidentiality towards third parties.

When modern methods of communications are employed, therefore, which for medical, scientific or administrative reasons involve the recording of data in such a way that they no longer remain under the direct control of the doctor, it is necessary to take all possible security measures to ensure the maintenance of confidentiality.

Under the pretext of better planning of health policy, of scientific research based on more reliable statistics, of more rapid access to medical records in case of accident, and of general rationalisation for the sake of efficiency, efforts are being made to gather together in data banks large amounts of information on individual patients. This involves the danger that these data will be recorded, examined and transmitted by third parties without the possibility of the patient concerned or his doctor judging the necessity for such actions or of monitoring the nature, the importance and the use of these data in individual cases.

General practitioners believe that personal data received by the doctor in the course of his professional duties should be released to a computerised data system accessible to third parties other than surgery or hospital staff, only when the following safeguards are applied:

(1) The permission of both the patient and his doctor should have been obtained.

(2) The patient should be able to obtain information on the nature and the implications of the data recorded about him, but that such information should only be transmitted through the doctor who supplied the data or, where appropriate, the doctor who is treating him.

(3) The patient in agreement with his doctor, should be able to correct or delete information appearing on the record.

(4) Safeguards should be applied to prevent abuse of the information or access by unauthorised persons.

(5) All personal information of a medical nature should be kept separate from other types of information accessible to persons other than the doctor.

(6) That the responsibility for the use of computerised medical data-system should rest exclusively with doctors.

The European Union of General Practitioners (UEMO) emphasises that all legislation should take into account the principles and conditions laid down above.

12   Resolutions of BMA annual representative meetings

The general control and direction of the policy and affairs of the British Medical Association is vested in the Representative Body. Six hundred doctors, representing the medical profession in the United Kingdom, meet annually to debate matters of concern to the profession. Some decisions of the meetings of the Representative Body on ethical matters are listed below:

AID

That this Meeting supports Council's efforts to secure a change in the law, so that a child born as a result of AID to which the husband of the mother has consented in writing, is recognised as legitimate from the time of confirmation of conception. (1979)

Certification

That this Meeting deplores the increased tendency to require specific diagnosis in non-statutory medical certificates. (1952)
That this Meeting strongly recommends practitioners not to issue "Duration Certificates" (ie certificates to insurance companies re the medical history of a person who has died soon after acceptance—without a medical report—for a Life Assurance). (1962—reaffirmed 1964 and 1983)

Child health service

That the care of the sick child remains primarily the responsibility of the general practitioner supported by his consultant colleagues. (1976)

Clinical teams

That the development of clinical teams must in no circumstances prejudice the ultimate responsibility of the doctor. (1979)

Code of conduct for patients

That the attention of the Government be drawn to the need for continuous education of the public, both in youth and adult life, in the constructive and responsible use of the National Health Service. (1956)

Confidentiality of medical records

Wherever practicable, and particularly where disclosure of information may have an adverse psychological effect upon the patient, the practitioner who compiled the record or, if he is not available, one nominated by the hospital authority for the purpose, should be consulted on the wisdom of disclosing to the patient all of the confidential information contained therein, and should take the opportunity of reviewing the notes before they leave the hospital. (1955)

That this Meeting agrees with the principle that specialists and general practitioners should not comply with requests from lay officials of local authorities for reports, as such requests should be made through the Medical Officer of Health (now the appropriate community physician). (1968)

That medical information should be absolutely confidential between doctor and patient and should only be divulged to para-medical workers working in direct professional relationship with the doctor. (1969)

In all medical records, information should be regarded as held for the specific purpose of the continuing care of the patient, and should not be used, without appropriate authorisation by the responsible clinician or the consent of the patient, for any other purpose. (1977)

That this Meeting insists that access to identifiable information held in medical records should be restricted to the author and the person clinically responsible for the patient during the episode for which the data was collected (or their successor) unless specifically authorised by the clinician in the interests of the patient. (1978)

That access to clinical data of previous episodes of illness be available to the clinicians having care of the patient, with the consent of the patient where it is practicable to obtain this. (1979)

That Association policy in relation to confidentiality of medical records should not preclude the exchange of information for any proper purpose between registered medical practitioners. (1979)

That this Meeting confirms that there is an essential continuing role for doctors trained in the fields of preventive and educational medicine, and that this can only benefit all individuals in the population if important information is shared freely, but with full precautions to maintain confidentiality between doctors practising curative and preventive medicine. (1980)

That no copy of a hospital specialist's reply to a GP patient referral should be sent to a non-medical third party without the knowledge and consent of the child's parent or guardian or without the agreement of the referring GP. (1980)

That Conference supports the recommendation of the General Medical Services Committee that copies of letters from consultant paediatricians to general practitioners about child patients referred to them should only be sent to other doctors where there is a specific clinical reason and that this should be to a named doctor. Routine distribution of copies of such letters should not occur. (1982)

Computerised medical records

That this meeting believes that no doctor should be party to the recording or holding of clinical information on any computer system which cannot completely safeguard the confidentiality of such information and requires Government to introduce adequate legislative safeguards, before the implementation of any further computer system. (1978)

That this Meeting considers that a comprehensive *statutory* code is essential for the protection of data-processing of medical records. (1982)

Declaration of Tokyo

That the Association endorses, in full, the Declaration of Tokyo 1975 of the WMA. (1979)

Euthanasia

That this Meeting affirms that the position of medical practitioners who are in conscience opposed to euthanasia must be fully protected in future legislation should it occur and that no legal obligation in this respect should be allowed to be imposed unilaterally on any member of the profession at any time. (1977)

Freedom to prescribe

That this Meeting protests in the strongest possible terms against any Government actions aimed at curtailing the freedom of a registered medical practitioner to prescribe—under suitable agreed safeguards—whether under the NHS or privately, whatever he thinks is best for his patient until and unless there is some absolutely overwhelming reason to the contrary which has been agreed between the profession as a whole and the Minister. (1956)

That this Representative Body will resist any attempt by Government to interfere with the doctor's right to prescribe the drug of his choice to his patient. (1976)

Industrial action

That this Meeting unequivocally condemns the kind of industrial action which increases the sum of human suffering. (1979)

Medical audit

That this Meeting instructs Council to investigate methods of audit within the profession and to report back. (1977)

Oral contraceptives

That this Meeting considers that the contraceptive pill should be available only on prescription by a registered medical practitioner. (1976—reaffirmed 1977)

Patients' access to case notes

That the medical profession must resist any legislation allowing patients access to their clinical case notes. (1980)

Press announcements of new drugs

That this Meeting deplores the publication in the popular press of extracts from medical articles and newspaper articles of an irresponsible character praising new drugs without illustrating any potential dangers. (1953)

92

Political and religious dissenters

That this Meeting condemns the practice of using medical men to certify political and religious dissenters as insane and to submit them to unnecessary investigation and treatment. (1973)

That this Representative Body deplores the continued abuse of medical skills and ethics for political ends in contravention of the principles of the Declaration of Geneva. (1976)

Professional independence

That this Meeting agrees that the policy of the Association shall be:—

(i) Freedom of the doctor to choose his patient.

(ii) Freedom of the patient to choose his doctor.

(iii) Freedom for the doctor in his clinical assessment and therapy.

(iv) That the doctor be entitled to a fee from his patient where the payment made by the State is considered by the profession to be inadequate for the services rendered.

(v) Freedom for the patient to avail himself of all or any relevant services available within the framework of the Welfare State. (1967)

Professions allied to medicine

That while there is no objection to the employment by most medical practitioners of radiographers for the purpose of taking films, the responsibility for the interpretation of such films must rest with a radiologist or other qualified medical practitioner. (1939)

That this Representative Body reaffirms that with proper arrangements for supervision by a consultant, access to hospital physiotherapy departments for urgent treatment should be available to family doctors where local circumstances demand it. (1965)

Television advertisements

That the televising of advertisements for pharmaceutical products, either directly or indirectly by the Science Survey type of programme or by fictitious doctors giving fictitious advice, would be prejudicial to the best interests of medical practice in this country. (1954)

Bibliography

Abortion, contraception and sterilisation

Abortion Act 1967. Chapter 87. London: HMSO, 1967.

BMA Committee on Therapeutic Abortion. Indications for termination of pregnancy. *Brit Med J* 1968; i: 171–5.

Department of Health and Social Security. *The use of fetuses and fetal material for research.* Report of the Advisory Group. London: HMSO, 1972. (Peel report.)

Committee on the Working of the Abortion Act. *Report.* Vol I–III. London: HMSO, 1974. (Lane report.) (Cmnd 5579-I, 5579-II.)

Seller M. Congenital abnormalities and selective abortions. *J Med Ethics* 1976; 2: 138–41.

Tunkel V. Abortion: how early, how late, and how legal? *Brit Med J* 1979; ii: 253–6.

Gardner R F. The ethics of abortion. *Practitioner* 1979; 223: 244–8.

Duncan S L B. Ethical problems in advising contraception and sterilisation. *Practitioner* 1979; 223: 237–42.

Anonymous. Late consequences of abortion. [Leader.] *Brit Med J* 1981; 282: 1564.

Consent to treatment

Garnham J C. Some observations on informed consent in non-therapeutic research. *J Med Ethics* 1975; 1: 138–45.

Anonymous. Valid parental consent. *Lancet* 1977; i: 1346–7.

Clothier C M. The law and the juvenile donor. *Lancet* 1977; i: 1356–7.

Skegg P D G. English law relating to experimentation on children. *Lancet* 1977; ii: 754–5.

Anonymous. Human experimentation: human rights. *Lancet* 1978; ii: 1352.

Vere D. Testing new drugs: the human volunteer. *J Med Ethics* 1978; 4: 81–3.

Anonymous. Consent to treatment. *Brit Med J* 1979; i: 1091–2.

Dunstan G R, Seller M J. *Consent in medicine: convergence and divergence in tradition.* London: King's Fund Centre, 1983.

Kirby M D. Informed consent: what does it mean? *J Med Ethics* 1983; 9: 69–75.

Genetics

Ellis H L. Parental involvement in the decision to treat spina bifida cystica. *Brit Med J* 1974; i: 369–72.

Newcastle Regional Hospital Board Working Party. Ethics of selective treatment of spina bifida. Report. *Lancet* 1975; i: 85–8.

Arnold A, Moseley R. Ethical issues arising from human genetics. *J Med Ethics* 1976; 2: 12–17.

Health and Safety Commission. *Genetic manipulation, regulations and guidance notes.* London: HMSO, 1978.

Ethics Advisory Board. *Health, education and welfare support of research involving human in vitro fertilisation and embryo transfer—report and conclusions.* Washington: US Government Printing Office, 1979. (017-040-00453-2.)

Harris J. Ethical problems in the management of some severely handicapped children. *J Med Ethics* 1981; 7: 117–24.

Seller M J. Ethical aspects of genetic counselling. *J Med Ethics* 1982; 8: 185–8.

British Medical Association. Interim report on human in-vitro fertilisation and embryo replacement and transfer. Report of Working Group on In-Vitro Fertilisation. Annual Report of Council 1983, Appendix VI. *Brit Med J* 1983; 286: 1594–5.

Industrial Action

Anonymous. Strikes in the National Health Service. *J Med Ethics* 1977; 3: 55.

Dworkin G. Strikes and the National Health Service: some legal and ethical issues. Commentary by P Zacharias. *J Med Ethics* 1977; 3: 76–82.

Royal College of Nursing. Code of professional conduct: a discussion document. *J Med Ethics* 1977; 3: 115–23.

Conference of Royal Medical Colleges of UK and BMA, Joint Working Party. Discussion document on ethical responsibilities of doctors practising in the National Health Service. *Brit Med J* 1977; i: 157–9.

Insemination, artificial

British Medical Association. Report of Panel on Human Artificial Insemination. Board of Science and Education. Annual Report of Council 1972, Appendix V. *Brit Med J* 1973; ii: 3–5.

Harrison R F, Wynn Williams G. Human artificial insemination. *Brit J Hosp Med* 1973; 9: 760–2.

Cusine D J. AID and the law. *J Med Ethics* 1975; 1: 39–41.

Cusine D J. Medico-legal aspects of AID. *IPPF Medical Bulletin* 1979; 13: 1–2.

Anonymous. Artificial insemination for all. *Brit Med J* 1979; ii: 458.

British Medical Association, ARM. Legitimacy for AID children. *Brit Med J* 1979; ii: 70.

Professional confidence

Home Office. *Report of the Committee on Privacy*. London: HMSO, 1972. (Younger report.) (Cmnd 5012.)

World Medical Association. Computers and confidentiality in medicine. *Brit Med J* 1973; ii: 290–3.

Barber B, Cohen R D, Kenny D J, Rowson J, Scholes M. Some problems of confidentiality in medical computing. *J Med Ethics* 1976; 2: 71–3.

Home Office. *Report of the Committee on Data Protection*. London: HMSO, 1978. (Lindop report.) (Cmnd 7341.)

Diamond B. Medical confidentiality and the law. *World Medicine* 1979; 14: 63–4.

Thompson I E. The nature of confidentiality. *J Med Ethics* 1979; 5: 57–64.

Pheby F H. Changing practice on confidentiality: a cause for concern. *J Med Ethics* 1982; 8: 12–24.

Terminal illness and death

British Medical Association. *The problem of euthanasia*. Report of a Special Panel of the Board of Science and Education. London: BMA, 1971.

Nicholson R. Should the patient be allowed to die? *J Med Ethics* 1975; 1: 5–9.

Campbell A G M. Moral dilemmas in the care of the dying. *Mimms Magazine* 1978; 2: 623–9.

Campbell A G M, Duff R S. Deciding the care of severely malformed or dying infants. *J Med Ethics* 1979; 5: 65–7.

Lawton, Lord Justice. Mercy killing: the judicial dilemma. *J Royal Soc Med* 1979; 72: 460–1.

Sweet T. Good or bad law. *J Royal Soc Med* 1979; 72: 461–4.

Rhoades J E. The right to die and the chance to live. *J Med Ethics* 1980; 6: 53–4.

Havard J D J. The legal threat to medicine. *Brit Med J* 1982; 284: 612–3.

Law Reform Commission of Canada. *Euthanasia, aiding suicide and cessation of treatment.* Report. Ottawa: Government Catalogue J31–40, 1983.

Transplantation

Jenet B. The donor doctor's dilemma: observations on the recognition and management of brain death. *J Med Ethics* 1975; 1: 63–6.

Knight B. Law and ethics in transplantation. *Practitioner* 1976; 216: 471–4.

Anonymous. Coroners and transplants. *Brit Med J* 1977; i: 1418.

Kennedy I. The donation and transplantation of kidneys: should the law be changed? *J Med Ethics* 1979; 5: 13–21.

Sells R A. Live organs from dead people. *J Royal Soc Med* 1979; 72: 109–17.

Department of Health and Social Security. *Cadaveric organs for transplantation.* A code of practice, including the diagnosis of brain death, drawn up and revised by a Working Party on behalf of the Health Departments of Great Britain and Northern Ireland. London: HMSO, 1983.

General

Ramsey P. *The patient as person.* New Haven and London: Yale University Press, 1970.

Taylor J Leahy. *The doctor and the law.* London: Pitman Medical and Scientific Publishing Co Ltd, 1970.

Veatch R M. *Case studies and medical ethics.* Cambridge Mass: Harvard University Press, 1977.

Duncan A S, Dunstan G R, Wellbourn R B. *Dictionary of Medical Ethics.* London: Darton, Longman and Todd, 1981.

Gillon R. The function of criticism. *Brit Med J* 1981; 283: 1633–9.

Sieghart P. Professional ethics—for whose benefit? *J Med Ethics* 1982; 8: 25–32.

British Medical Association. *The occupational physician.* London: BMA, 1982.

Association of British Pharmaceutical Industries. *Data sheet compendium 1983–84.* London: Datapharm Publications, 1983.

General Medical Council. *Professional conduct and discipline: fitness to practise.* London: GMC, 1983.

Mason J K, McCall R A. *Law and medical ethics.* London: Butterworths, 1983.

Index

pline" August 1983 p49 8.10

AID *see* INSEMINATION, Artificial by Donor

ALTERNATIVE MEDICAL CARE *see also* INTRA-PROFESSIONAL RELATIONS

Abortion, conscientious objection p59 10.3, 10.4

Industrial action by non-medically qualified people p35 5.2

Referral of patients p17 2.9—2.11

ARMED FORCES

Volunteers in experiments p19 2.14

ARMED FORCES MEDICAL OFFICERS

Confidentiality p24 2.33

Doctors in specialised communities p23 2.30

Ethical responsibilities p23 2.32

Interrogation and punishment p24 2.35

Monitoring of volunteers trained in techniques of resistance to interrogation p45 6.22

Servicemen's families p24 2.34

Signing certification of fitness p52 8.24

ARTIFICIAL FEEDING *see* FEEDING, Artificial

ARTIFICIAL INSEMINATION BY DONOR (AID) *see* INSEMINATION, Artificial

ASSAULT *see* CONSENT TO TREATMENT

ASSIGNMENT OF PATIENTS *see under* PATIENTS

ASSOCIATION OF BRITISH PHARMACEUTICAL INDUSTRIES

Code of Practice for the Assessment of Licensed Medicines in General Practice p31, 4.5

ASSURANCE

Life, examinations p25 3.1; p25 3.3, 3.4

Medical reports after death British Medical Association ARM decisions "Duration Certificates" ch12 p89

100

ATTENDANCE UPON COLLEAGUES *see under* DOCTOR(S)

AUDIT *see* MEDICAL AUDIT

BELGIUM

Ethical code p42 6.6

BILLS, Parliament

Euthanasia p64 10.29

BLOOD TRANSFUSION *see* JEHOVAH'S WITNESSES

BONE MARROW TRANSPLANTATION *see under* TISSUE TRANSPLANTATION

BRAIN DEATH

Conference of Medical Royal Colleges and their Faculties Reports. October 1976, January 1979 p65 10.34; ch11 p81

Doctors qualifications for deciding brain death p61 10.14

Termination of artificial support p65 10.34

Unpaired organs, transplantation p61 10.14

BRITISH ASSOCIATION OF SOCIAL WORKERS

Ethical code p41 5.27, 5.28

BRITISH MEDICAL ASSOCIATION

ARM ethical decisions p10; ch12 p89

Central Ethical Committee p9

Confidentiality p12 1.6(4); p15 1.19(c) *see also* p30 4.1—4.14

Formation p9

Intra-professional disagreements, BMA ethical machinery p54 8.36—8.38

Research ethical committees model constitution p31 4.6

CANVASSING

p51 8.21

CERTIFICATES AND STATEMENTS

p51 8.22—8.24

CERTIFICATION

British Medical Association ARM decisions ch12 p89

101

103

104

106

108